MRCGP: Preparation and Passing

Edited by

John J Ferguson TD FRCGP

Medical Director
Prescription Pricing Authority
Newcastle-upon-Tyne

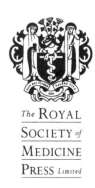

The ROYAL
SOCIETY *of*
MEDICINE
PRESS *Limited*

© 2000 Royal Society of Medicine Press Ltd
1 Wimpole Street, London W1G 0AE, UK
207 Westminster Road, Lake Forest, IL, 60045, USA

British Library Cataloguing in Publication Data
A catalogue record for this book is available from the British Library

ISBN 1-85315-468-7

Phototypeset by Phoenix Photosetting, Chatham, Kent

Printed in Great Britain by Bell and Bain Ltd, Glasgow

MRCGP: Preparation and Passing

NHS Staff Libr~

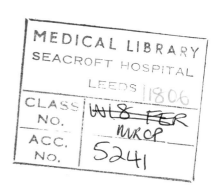

▶ Contents

▶ List of Contributors

Rifat A. Atun
28 Lincoln Avenue
London

Tim Ballard
The Old School Surgery
Great Bedwyn
Marlborough, Wilts

Eleanor Brown
Chief Executive
South Lambeth Primary Care Group
Greenvale, South London

Yvonne H Carter
Professor of General Practice and Primary Care
St Bartholomew's and London School of Medicine and Dentistry
Queen Mary & Westfield College
London

John Chisholm
Head, NHS GP's Division
British Medical Association
BMA House
London

Sandra Eldridge
Queen Mary and Westfield College University of London
St Bartholomew's and the Royal London School of Medicine and Dentistry
Department of General Practice and Primary Care
Medical Sciences
London

Maggie Falshaw
Queen Mary and Westfield College University of London
St Bartholomew's and the Royal London School of Medicine and Dentistry
Department of General Practice and Primary Care
Medical Sciences
London

John J Ferguson
Medical Director
Prescription Pricing Authority
Bridge House
Newcastle-upon-Tyne

Nigel Holmes
The Group Practice
Bengal Road
Bulford Camp
Salisbury, Wilts

Neil Jackson
St Bartholomew's and the Royal London School of Medicine and Dentistry
Department of General Practice and Primary Care
Medical Sciences
London

Margaret D Murray
14 Roughwood Close
Watford
Herts

Peter Orton
Matching Parsonage Farm
Newmans End
Matching
Essex

Gerard Panting
Head of Policy and External Relations
Medical Protection Society
London

Michael Pringle
School of Community Health Sciences
Division of General Practice
University Hospital
Queen's Medical Centre
Nottingham

Bashir Qureshi
Transcultural Medicine
Hounslow West Middlesex

John Schofield
Elsenham Surgery
Elsenham
Bishops Stortford
Hertfordshire

David Smalley
Nuffield House
The Stow
Essex

Richard Styles
Whitchurch Surgery
Bell Street
Whitchurch
Hampshire

Tim Swanwick
Vine House Health Centre
Abbots Langley
Hertfordshire

Peter Tate
The Clock House
High Street
Culham
Abingdon
Oxfordshire

Mike Thirlwall
Meadowcroft Surgery
Jackson Road
Aylesbury, Bucks

▶ Preface

Most young doctors entering British general practice want to take the MRCGP examination. All the evidence suggests that at the end of vocational training or shortly thereafter is the best time.

Most MRCGP candidates attend some form of preparation course. Sometimes it is included within their vocational training scheme and sometimes as a separate course. The object of a successful course is to educate and inform, and inform, and to take away the fear of the unknown.

This book is based on the highly successful five-day pre-MRCGP course held at the Royal Society of Medicine in London. I am most grateful to all those lecturers and MRCGP Examiners who have contributed to the success of the course, and who have so generously summarised their presentations for this book.

The first part of this book highlights the issues facing general practice at the start of the new millennium, along with information on important topics such as practice management, audit and prescribing.

The second part of this book is a detailed analysis of the MRCGP examination and all its component parts, and provides clear advice on how to best prepare for this examination in its current modular format.

I am most grateful for the assistance of Lynne Davis, Sarah Bayer, and the staff of the RSM Press and Naughton Project Management who have facilitated the production of this book so expeditiously.

Dr John J Ferguson
September 2000

Further Reading

Royal College of General Practitioners (1990) *Examination for Membership of the Royal College of General Practitioners (MRCGP). Occasional Paper 46.* London RCGP

Tombeson P, Wakeford R (1989) Why do trainees take the membership examination? *Journal of the Royal College of General Practitioners*, 39: 168–171

Lancet (1990) Examining the Royal College's examinations. Editorial, 335: 443

Godlee F (1991) MRCGP: examining the exam. *BMJ* 303: 235–238

MRCP Enquiries

Examination Department
The Royal College of General Practitioners
Princes Gate
Hyde Park
London
SW7 1PU

Tel: 0207 581 3232
Fax: 0207 225 3047 or 0207 584 3165
E-mail: *exams@rcgp.org.uk*

Information and news about the examination, which may be of interest to candidates is posted electronically on the College's Internet website:

http://www.recgp.org.uk

▶ 1

General Practice – Academic and Training Issues

Neil Jackson

Introduction

Postgraduate education and training for general practice is managed in the United Kingdom within the Postgraduate Deaneries of Medical and Dental Education by Directors (or Deans) of Postgraduate General Practice Education (DsPGPE) through their educational networks of Associate Directors (or Deans), course organisers, GP tutors and GP trainers.

DsPGPE have increasingly complex roles within the NHS education and training system and their line of accountability is ultimately to the Secretary of State for Health, through the Postgraduate Dean and the Director of Education and Training in the relevant Regional Office of the NHS Executive.

The Government's White Paper (Secretary of State for Health 1997) highlights the key principle of quality in the new NHS. Quality in the new NHS can only be promoted by a system of service delivery and development which is supported and informed by appropriate education and training, and research and development, i.e. a 'three systems approach' (Jackson 1999).

Within the Education and Training system in the NHS, increasingly high standards of general practice have been promoted by a number of key organisations and bodies including the Joint Committee on Postgraduate Training for General Practice (JCPTGP), the Royal College of General Practitioners (RCGP) and the General Practice Committee of the BMA (GPC), as well as DsPGPE and their educational networks. However, there is now a recognition that GP vocational training is in need of enhanced development to ensure that future GPs are 'fit for purpose' in terms of quality service provision in a modernised system of primary care.

The establishment of Primary Care Groups/Trusts (PCGs/PCTs) and the agenda for clinical governance will have profound implications for established GPs, including professional revalidation and a new system of Continuing Professional Development (CPD) to maintain the balance between personal and professional fulfilment and employability. Undoubtedly the need for education and training to support service provision in the NHS has never been greater.

Vocational training for general practice – present state and historial background

The NHS General Practice Vocational Training Regulations were established in 1979 and came into operation in early 1980. A transition phase then followed and from 1982 three years full-time employment (or part-time equivalent) was required to satisfy the Regulations for prescribed experience, that is at least one year as a trainee general practitioner (GP Registrar) and the remainder in educationally approved posts as detailed in the Regulations. Since then the constructed three-year vocational training programme has typically consisted of two years of specialist hospital posts at senior house officer level and twelve months undertaken as a GP Registrar in an approved postgraduate training practice. Inevitably, the teaching skills of GP trainers have become more highly developed since the advent of formal vocational training for general practice, and the concept of quality teaching in protected time is now well established. In addition, the postgraduate GP training practice has become a specialised learning environment which now recognises the need for a multiprofessional/multidisciplinary approach to education and training.

Since 1990 (JCPTGP, GMSC and RCGP 1990) there has been a shift in emphasis towards a competence-based approach to vocational training. GP Registrars are now required to achieve minimum standards of competence by successful completion of a summative assessment programme. This was introduced on a voluntary basis from September 1996 (Conference of Postgraduate Advisers in General Practice 1995). However, summative assessment became legally mandatory following the revision of the NHS GP Vocational Training Regulations in 1997.

Since its inception the summative assessment programme has consisted of four separate modules or components, all of which must be successfully completed: a written test (multiple-choice questions and extended matching questions); a written submission (audit presentation); a videotape of actual consultations with patients to demonstrate competence with reference to consultation skills; and a structured trainer's report (completed by the GP trainer towards the end of the GP Registrar training year).

It is important to note that the summative assessment programme is currently in a state of development. The written submission will in future include other forms of written material as an alternative to an audit. Consultation skills will also be tested by a simulated surgery using standardised patients as an alternative to videotaped consultations.

The majority of GP Registrars sit and pass the membership of the Royal College of General Practitioners (MRCGP) examination in addition to successfully completing the summative assessment programme. The examination has been thoroughly researched and developed and there is now an increasing commitment to testing communication and consultation skills. The MRCGP as an examination has done much to raise the standards of general practice. This also applies to the panel of examiners, many of whom are Associate DsPGPE, course organisers or experienced GP trainers from established postgraduate training practices.

Future priorities for general practice education and training

Development of GP vocational training

As from April 2000 in England and Wales the funding for GP vocational training will be transferred from the General Medical Services (GMS) budget to the Medical and Dental Education Levy (MADEL) (Field *et al* 2000).

(NB: In Scotland GP Registrars salaries were transferred from health boards to the Scottish Council for Postgraduate Medical and Dental Education in April 1998. In Northern Ireland the GMS to MADEL transfer from the GMS budget to the Northern Ireland Council for Postgraduate Medicine and Dental Education was effected in April 1999.)

The GMS to MADEL transfer of funding will be managed within Postgraduate Medical and Dental Deaneries by DsPGPE and the implications are significant in terms of the development of GP vocational training. The Committee of General Practice Education Directors (COGPED) defined a set of core principles in 1999 to underpin the GMS to MADEL transfer and the enhanced arrangements for the management of GP training and these are summarised as follows:

▶ Robust, credible, fair selection procedures for GPVTS SHOs/GP Registrars with equal opportunities and effective screening of problem trainees.

▶ Equitable distribution of GPVTS SHOs/GP Registrars to meet future workforce needs.

▶ Efficient use of resources by DsPGPE with managerial accountability.

▶ Measurable quality outcomes.

▶ Satisfying GP Registrars personal and educational needs.

▶ Meeting GP trainer needs, i.e. providing indemnity cover for training through the Deanery and the enhancement of teaching and educational skills through CPD.

Future strategic priorities for the development of GP vocational training will also include the strengthening of training programmes by improving the GP focus of VTS SHO posts; monitoring study leave arrangements for GP trainees; strengthening the Pre-Registration House Officer GP placement scheme and the provision of enhanced support for doctors in training to prevent and effectively manage poor clinical performance.

Post-vocational training support

It is well recognised that there is a need to develop a framework for Higher Professional Education (HPE) for GP Registrars completing basic vocational training. Many recently vocationally trained GPs would benefit from an additional one or two years of training spent as a 'Senior GP Registrar' in an approved learning practice to develop research and teaching skills, to undertake a Master's degree course or to develop clinical specialist skills. A period of HPE in a supportive learning environment would do much to prepare and develop the modern GP required for the future.

The concept of higher professional education is relevant to all new GPs following the completion of vocational training and includes young principals, non-principals, salaried doctors and retainers. The important issue is to provide on-going educational support at a crucial time in a young GP's career to enhance both competence and confidence.

There is also a need to improve the provision of educational support in general for non-principal GPs who have been a sadly neglected group in the past. DsPGPE and their educational networks are now actively addressing this issue.

General Practitioners in established practice – Continuing Professional Development

With the advent of Primary Care Groups/Primary Care Trusts (PCGs/PCTs) in the new NHS, the role of established GPs has become pivotal. The emphasis on clinical governance as the means by which organisations ensure the provision of clinical care by making individuals accountable for setting, maintaining and monitoring performance standards will require all GPs to maintain a high standard of performance and become 'lifelong' learners in the NHS by a process of appropriate CPD. This will be set in a multiprofessional/multidisciplinary context in primary care. Practice professional development plans (PPDPs) and individual GP personal development plans (PDPs) will be implemented and monitored by the clinical governance leads of PCGs/PCTs and DsPGPE. PDPs are crucial to the professional revalidation of individual GPs and will need to be clearly linked to PPDPs and the clinical governance agenda within individual GP practices and PCGs/PCTs.

Established GPs will also require appropriate and effective mechanisms of educational support to prevent and manage poor clinical performance.

Academic and training issues – the primary care context

Vocational training for general practice and continuing education for established GPs has become increasingly set within a multiprofessional/multidisciplinary context. There is also gathering momentum in primary care for the medical and nursing professions, together with professions allied to medicine (PAMs), to work and learn together from undergraduate through to postgraduate levels. Along with this has come a shift in emphasis from the health of individuals to the health of populations. This is now reflected in the increasingly community orientated undergraduate teaching programmes for medical students, with some medical schools delivering up to 20% of their curricula in the community.

Postgraduate GP training practices and university-linked practices for general practice undergraduate teaching are evolving into the learning practices of the future, where health care professionals learn and develop together as a team in a primary care setting (Carter et al 1998). Such practices are also managing the interfaces between education and training and service provision and research and development. This in turn will promote higher standards of patient care.

The learning practice model can be adapted for all GP practices within PCG/PCT boundaries and this in part can be facilitated by DsPGPE through their educational networks.

DsPGPE are also actively encouraging each PCG/PCT to develop an education and training strategy for the benefit of its constituent members at practice organisational and individual health care professional levels. It is essential for PCGs/PCTs to take charge of their own education and training agendas and this should also embrace workforce planning issues as well as ensuring effective working and learning for all staff members and teams across professional and organisational boundaries (Carter and Jackson 1999).

References

Carter Y, Jackson N (1999). Primary care groups: criteria, expectations and education and training issues. *Education for General Practice* **10**: 411–416.

Carter Y, Jackson N, Barnfield A (1998). The learning practice: a new model for primary health teams. *Education for General Practice* **9**: 182–197.

Conference of Postgraduate Advisers in General Practice (1995). *Summative Assessment*. Universities of the UK.

Field S, Allen K, Jackson N, *et al* (2000). Vocational training: the dawn of a new era? *Education for General Practice* **11**: 1–8.

Jackson N (1999). Quality in the new NHS – the role of education and training in General Practice and Primary Care. *Education for General Practice* **10**: 6–8.

Secretary of State for Health (1997). *The New NHS*. London: HMSO.

►2

The General Practitioners Committee's View

John Chisholm

The General Practitioners Committee (GPC) of the British Medical Association (BMA) represents all National Health Service (NHS) general practitioners, whether or not they are members of the BMA, whether they are principals or non-principals, independent contractors or salaried, providing general medical services or personal medical services, whether in training for general practice or already fully trained. The GPC is recognised by the Government as the sole negotiating body for general practice.

A year ago, I announced that the GPC was initiating a policy review – a thorough and extensive process of mapping out possible futures and initiating widespread debate inside and outside general practice; a GP-led approach to defining our own agenda for the future, in part as a response to the constant changes in the NHS that are imposed by Government.

We are now well into that process. In February, every GP in the UK was sent Chris Mihill's *Shaping Tomorrow: Issues Facing General Practice in the New Millennium.* It set out the key strengths of general practice, the problems and threats that confront us, and possible solutions for the next decade. It was intended to stimulate and inform a wide process of discussion, including local medical meetings throughout the country and our first ever GPC Conference in Harrogate on 15 March. That conference included workshops and question and answer sessions on key issues affecting our future and contributions by the Prime Minister, the Secretary of State for Health and a number of leading thinkers about health care, and provided an exciting platform for debating the ferment of ideas about the future for general practice.

The consultation process on which the GPC has embarked is intended to culminate in policy decisions that will underpin our future negotiating agenda, promote and strengthen general practice in the new millennium, protect its fundamental characteristics and its pivotal role, embrace appropriate change and ensure a service of which we and our patients can be proud.

A year ago, GPs were being criticised for their conservatism. But we are not hostile to change. We have never been afraid to take on new ideas, new challenges and new ways of working. We embrace change constantly, whether it is in the field of clinical practice, service delivery or postgraduate education. Primary care teams, an extended range of services provided in general practice, premises development, vocational training and out-of-hours cooperatives are all examples of changes which have been initiated from within general practice.

As we enter a new millennium, we need to map out and embrace further change, to strengthen and make the most of our GP-led approach to defining an agenda for the future. We need to take stock of what being a GP should mean in the years ahead, what we need from Government and what we expect of ourselves.

The publication of Mihill's book and the debates at our Harrogate conference could not have been better timed in terms of demonstrating that we were indeed eager to take a constructive and positive approach to the improvement of health care. The very next week, the Chancellor of the Exchequer announced a substantial addition to NHS funding, and the Prime Minister laid down five challenges for the NHS and announced the establishment of six Modernisation Action Teams in England.

The NHS spending announcement gave substance to the pledge the Prime Minister had made earlier in the year. There is to be a 35% real terms rise in funding over five years, a 6.1% real terms average increase over the next four years, and an immediate injection in the present financial year of an additional £2 billion. By 2003–2004, health care spending in the UK will have risen to 7.6% of GDP – a very substantial rise that cannot but be welcomed as an immense opportunity for the health service. It should help address many of the problems of the NHS, if it is spent wisely, but it will not answer all problems. We must not forget that we will still be spending less than many comparable developed countries, and it remains entirely appropriate that over the next year the BMA is conducting a review of UK health care funding, looking at public expectations, wants and needs and the resources and funding arrangements required.

The five Blair challenges – the partnership and performance challenges, the challenge for the professions, the patient care challenge and the challenge on prevention – have in England led to the creation of six Modernisation Action Teams, with patient care being addressed in relation to both speed of access and patient empowerment. Those teams involve a broad coalition of health care professionals, managers, civil servants and patients, and should herald a more inclusive method of policy formation, not just in relation to the creation of the National Plan for the New NHS, but thereafter also. I believe we should welcome the fact that senior BMA members are involved in that process. Whilst some have pointed to the undoubted risks of such close involvement, I would far rather that the GPC and the BMA were closely involved than that they were excluded.

However, one of the early tasks for the Committee and for the profession will be to address the impact and the implementation of the National Plan. In Scotland and Wales, GPs have a different and less overtly inclusive method of considering how the additional resources should be spent in their countries. Meanwhile GPs in Northern Ireland continue to experience the frustration of the policy vacuum created by the uncertainties surrounding the Northern Ireland Assembly. I hope that the restoration of devolved government will now allow rapid implementation of the reforms the profession has been suggesting, including the establishment of Primary Care Cooperatives, which have much in common with English Primary Care Groups (PCGs). In Scotland, the continued exclusion of GPs from secondary care commissioning and the failure of the Joint Investment Fund concept are enduring causes for concern.

The implementation of PCGs has been undermined by inadequate funding. From the start, there has been under-resourcing at every stage: too little money for preparation, too little for the continuing costs, too little for organisational development, education and training, too little for management costs and payments to board members, too little investment in the information systems essential for strategic planning and clinical governance.

All the primary care organisations in Great Britain – PCGs in England, Local Health Groups in Wales and Local Health Care Cooperatives in Scotland – have continued to experience difficulties because of underfunding and budgetary pressures, resulting from generic drug shortages and price rises, the need to fund the nurses' pay award, and the additional costs of new treatments of proven benefit. However, the GPC has corrected a longstanding injustice by negotiating the superannuation of allowances paid to PCT and PCG board members, and is also currently involved in negotiations to end the wholly unjustifiable exclusion of self-employed GP locums from the NHS Superannuation Scheme.

Even now that more money has been passed on to Primary Care Groups and Trusts, it has been mostly swallowed up by previous overspends and by the hospital service. It is essential that a substantial proportion of the additional £2 billion available in the current financial year does fund primary care development; in the first year of the new structures many proposals for such development, for service shifts and for intermediate care have had to be put on ice. GPs' cynicism and demoralisation will increase if the energy and vision they have put into making the new structures work is undermined by a lack of the resources needed to transform their vision into reality.

The first year of PCGs has seen large numbers of proposals for progression to Primary Care Trust status put forward by Health Authorities, Community Trusts or PCGs. The great majority of these proposals have not gone forward in April 2000, but there will be a further group of PCGs that make the transition in October 2000 and a significant number in April 2001. The GPC believes that the overwhelming majority of local GPs should approve a proposal before it goes forward. Whilst most GPs are realistic about the inevitability of progression from PCGs to PCTs, they rightly feel that they should have a major say in the pace of change. It is important that they are fully informed about the nature of a proposal through the consultation process before final decisions are made. Progression will and should take place at different rates in different areas. PCTs should build on success rather than grow out of failure, and PCT proposals should demonstrate both success as a PCG and the added value that will accrue from a move to Trust status.

There has been much consternation about the approval of the Southend PCT in the face of local GP opposition, and the GPC both lobbied politicians and sought expert legal advice to see whether the approval could be overturned. The reality is, alas, that there were no legal grounds for doing so, and the advice we received has been issued to all Local Medical Committees, for Southend may not be the last PCT to be approved despite GP opposition demonstrated in a ballot. But there is another reality that Ministers should bear in mind. GPs are a fundamental part of the local health care economy. Their goodwill and application is vital to the success of any health care reorganisation, and their wishes must not be set aside in a cavalier manner.

Another area of recent concern has been out-of-hours care. The doctors who have benefited least from the negotiations concluded in 1995 have been those in geographically isolated areas. In the last financial year in England, £2 million of the out-of-hours development fund was set aside and allocated to help those doctors establish schemes above the level of their individual practices. For months, we pressed the Department to continue that targeted allocation this year. Yet we were not told until mid-April of its replacement by a capitation-based allocation as a result of a unilateral decision by the Department, without any prior consultation. That crass decision threatens the quality of patient care in rural areas, is the antithesis of family-friendly policy, and has caused great anger throughout the profession. Geographically isolated out-of-hours services must be protected.

The other out-of-hours issue that has caused concern is the establishment of an out-of-hours review in England. We are represented on the review reference group and have met the review team, but are concerned lest the outcome undermines in any way the high quality, cost-effective out-of-hours care that has been developed in recent years, to the benefit of patients, doctors and their families. The public rightly expects to be treated by alert, competent GPs. We are determined that these advantages should not be lost or diminished.

The jury is still out on NHS Direct, the nurse-led telephone triage service. The second interim evaluation of the first wave sites has not yet established whether the service, which is undoubtedly popular with the public, is improving health outcomes and the appropriateness with which people use the NHS, is safeguarding other parts of the NHS and providing value for money. As yet, there is no evidence that NHS Direct is having an important effect on overall demand for accident and emergency or ambulance services, or that it is reducing the demands on general practice. The evaluation must be continued until there are clear answers to all these questions. Similarly, the place of walk-in centres in the panoply of NHS provision needs to be rigorously evaluated. However, LMCs, PCGs and GP cooperatives need to be constructively involved in these developments rather than stand aside, so as to ensure properly integrated care.

This year has been overshadowed by revelations concerning the tragic and terrible events in Hyde, where a callous and evil man who happened to be a doctor betrayed his patients, their relatives and his profession. Whilst it is Harold Shipman who is guilty, not British general practice, and whilst the vast majority of doctors are honest and trustworthy and deliver high-quality care, it is appropriate that there should be a full enquiry into this appalling case and that lessons should be learnt, in the interests of patients and the profession. The GPC is actively involved in preparing evidence for the Laming Enquiry and the Home Office review, considering regulatory changes and discussing current mechanisms and new proposals for handling underperformance. The outcome from this work must be proportionate and fit for purpose. We cannot countenance a situation where trustworthy GPs and consultants are constantly under suspicion. Those doctors are of enormous value to their patients and deliver high-quality care and the health service cannot run without them.

Another area in which the GPC has taken the lead, through constructive partnership with the Royal College of General Practitioners and other general practice organisations, is in developing proposals for revalidation, designed to demonstrate to the public that their doctors are providing a high standard of care and remain up to date and fit to practise.

In January, all GPs in the UK, and patient groups, NHS organisations and other professional bodies, were sent two documents, *Revalidation for Clinical General Practice* and *Good Medical Practice for General Practitioners*, which describe what is expected of a GP. These documents contain provisional proposals and will evolve in the light of consultation, but so far they have been well received. They build on the lead taken by the GPC and the RCGP throughout most of the past decade in developing proposals for reaccreditation and recertification. However, the precise nature of revalidation will crucially depend on the resources and time available for the process. The GPC will consider the consultation document, which the GMC has published recently, and will work closely with the RCGP in responding on behalf of general practice.

Revalidation has to complement clinical governance within quality assurance. Shortly, the Department of Health will publish its response to the English Chief Medical Officer's discussion document *Supporting Doctors, Protecting Patients*. We responded to that document jointly with the RCGP and the Joint Committee on Postgraduate Training for General Practice, and had particular concerns about the nature of the appraisal process and the concept of Assessment and Support Centres. However, we wish to see effective mechanisms for handling underperformance, and were pleased to see the CMO acknowledging that remediation requires public funding.

Whilst the General Medical Council has been understandably criticised about its communications and the slowness of its fitness to practise procedures, it has listened to those criticisms. It has appointed a Director of Communications, has secured the power to appoint non-GMC members, both medical and lay, to its fitness to practise committees, and is setting performance targets which will see a dramatic reduction over the next year in the time taken to address complaints. These measures should restore confidence in the General Medical Council and ensure that it properly fulfils its paramount duty to protect patients. Professionally led regulation is immensely valuable, and the GMC needs not only constructive criticism but also the profession's support for the changes it is making. Votes of no confidence in the GMC are too easily construed as a lack of confidence in professionally led regulation itself, which I believe is the hallmark of a profession.

For many years the need for NHS services has outstripped resources – a situation as unacceptable to the medical profession as it is to the public and the Government. That is why the increased NHS funding that has been announced is so welcome. That is why GPs are ready to meet the challenge of modernisation. The NHS must be developed in a way which will meet the aspirations of patients and the public whilst also being fair to health care professionals. To achieve both aims, it is essential that public expectations are not raised beyond a level which can be met reasonably within the resources available.

GPs welcome the Government's recognition of the crucial importance of primary care within the NHS. There is a need to let go of outdated responsibilities and mechanisms. But there is a need also to reward work and responsibility fully. The outcome should be an NHS which provides enhanced patient care whilst also delivering increased job satisfaction and better working conditions for those who work within it.

The GPC has identified a number of areas where radical change and service developments are possible, both to improve services for patients and to provide satisfaction for GPs as part of the primary care team. These include quality, skill mix, information management and technology, patient-friendly services, intermediate care and recruitment and retention.

All professionals in primary care wish to provide a high quality service for their patients. Continuing professional development (CPD) and clinical decisions informed by best practice are essential. Demands on GPs' time currently prevent full participation in CPD, in audit and in reflective practice. It is crucial that protected time for these is available for all doctors.

Time is also required for clinical care, as there is clear evidence that the length of the consultation has a direct relationship to a high quality outcome. To deliver that time for a longer GP–patient dialogue during the consultation, which both doctors and patients want, other members of the team will need to undertake some of the work traditionally done by the GP.

Whereas in the past, GPs personally dealt with all conditions presented to them, it is now recognised that this is neither tenable nor appropriate. Other health professionals can often play a more effective part. Nurses have a role in triage, prescribing and chronic disease management. Pharmacists have a role in prescribing advice and the management of self-limiting illness. Physiotherapists have a role in rehabilitation. However, it is axiomatic that the GP remains the diagnostician, the clinical generalist and the ultimate risk manager within the team.

Better use of the skills of all the members of the primary care team can and should be made now. However, there is also a longer-term agenda of planning for future workforce requirements. Those who imagine that nurses can somehow instantly solve the problems of the health service by taking over all that GPs do are deluded; doctors and nurses have distinct but complementary roles, and allied to this there is a major shortage of nurses as well as of GPs.

The huge advances in information management and technology will enable significant progress in disseminating effective medical information to doctors, patients and the public about clinical issues, and also facilitate the communication of personal health information between professionals and to individual patients. Further Government investment in state-of-the-art technology is required to take advantage of the improved efficiencies that electronic communications can provide.

The GPC has concluded a satisfactory agreement with the Department of Health in which GPs will pay nothing whatsoever for the installation, connection and 24-hour-a-day use of NHS Net – an NHS Net that has been significantly improved through negotiation. Project Connect will be totally free to GPs. Obviously the full potential of such connectivity will only be realised once encrypted personal health information can be sent over the network in a way that fully protects patient confidentiality.

The way patients access medical services has changed significantly over the last 20 years, and the profession recognises that the traditional general practice model is no longer always appropriate. The GPC is willing to explore alternative models of provision better to reflect the needs of patients, and also it sees potential in increased patient involvement and empowerment.

The GPC shares the current enthusiasm for the intermediate care concept, including its potential to deliver improved rehabilitation and convalescence, and is keen to discuss how appropriate alternative models of service and premises provision might be developed.

The modernisation of primary care requires an increase in the number of professionals if the quality of patient care is to be enhanced and, not least, an increase in the numbers of GPs. The UK has fewer doctors per head than any other comparably developed country. General practice must become an attractive option for those at the start of their careers, as well as encouraging those already in practice to continue with enthusiasm and dedication. This requires family-friendly policies, a full occupational health service for GPs and their staff, and improved, relevant training of sufficient duration for young doctors to feel confident in their craft.

General practice is a fundamental part of health care. At its centre is the care provided to people who are ill or believe themselves to be ill, and at its heart a doctor–patient relationship founded on mutual trust and personal attention focused on the individual.

General practice will and must continue to have a distinctive and enduring place in health care. Whilst specialists confirm the presence of serious disease, the task of the general practitioner is to exclude its presence. GPs accept uncertainty, explore probability and marginalise danger. That work of a clinical generalist, that diagnostic task, is both quite different from and no less intellectually and professionally demanding than the diagnostic task of the specialist, which is to reduce uncertainty, explore possibility and marginalise error.

In the UK, general practice is highly valued by most patients. Like their doctors, they realise that knowing the person who has the disease is as important as knowing the disease the person has. Its cost-effectiveness and efficiency, in terms of costs for given outcomes, are founded on the patient list, responsibility for a defined population, the lifelong medical record and access to clinical generalists who coordinate care and decide whether referral to a specialist is required. That gatekeeper role is exercised with discretion: some 90% of health care episodes that come to the notice of the NHS are handled entirely within primary care. These concepts underpin the British model of general practice are envied by other countries, commended by the World Health Organisation, and rightly have an enduring value.

There is significant international research evidence, most notably from Barbara Starfield, about the importance of family medicine. Those systems that give the right of referral to GPs with a gatekeeper function are more efficient in their use of a nation's wealth for health care, have lower health care costs and better health outcomes. In other words, health systems that have a strong emphasis on primary care and a strong family doctor service make better use of the resources applied to health care and also provide better health outcomes than those systems with less emphasis on primary care.

However, we need to develop a modern, efficient and high-quality primary care service for the 21st century. It makes sense to embrace and shape change, rather than have it imposed. GPs are willing to let go of outdated responsibilities. They are willing to look at radical change. Family doctors are willing to play a full part in determining how best to modernise the NHS to the benefit of patients, the public and health care professionals. But in identifying what can be changed, we must also define what is special, central and enduring about our role as general practitioners. Then we must work to persuade and convince others to share our vision of a better future.

▶3

General Practice – The RCGP's View

Michael Pringle

Introduction

This chapter reviews five key issues for British general practice at the start of the twenty-first century.

▶ The extent to which the health services in Britain, both within and outside the National Health Service, will crucially influence the range and level of service patients receive.

▶ The workforce, since funding cannot be used effectively and efficiently without sufficient numbers of skilled staff – doctors, nurses and other members of the primary care team.

▶ Vocational training, which is creaking in its 1979 straight jacket and is a clear case for reform.

▶ Challenges to the regulation of the profession as part of a national debate on quality of care, patient expectations and our capacity to meet those expectations.

▶ Access to care. This has been the real battlefield of the past three years and is likely to continue to be so for the immediate future.

Health service funding

Every society has to make difficult decisions on how health care will be funded. In the nineteenth century the consensus was that health care was a personal responsibility. However, a few enlightened employers recognised that health care for workers, and sometimes their families, was a good investment. As soon as skills rise and are prized – and thus the workforce is not easily replenished – the case for collective responsibility for health care grows.

In the last century we saw, through, for example, Lloyd George's National Insurance scheme and then the creation of the National Health Service, an increasing recognition that health care could not be left to market forces. Almost every Western country then adopted this paradigm. The major exception has been the United States of America, but even there Medicaid and Medicare have offered national safety nets for the elderly and the poor.

Once the State becomes involved in health care, health care becomes politicised. As medicines and interventions become more complex, risky and expensive this is probably inevitable. One key element that becomes politicised is the proportion of national wealth that will be dedicated to health care.

As Figure 3.1 shows, Britain spends 6.5% of its gross domestic product (GDP) on the NHS and private health care, whereas even the state sector in the United States spends 7% (and 14% overall). To rise to the level of France or Germany, we would need to spend half as much again on health care.

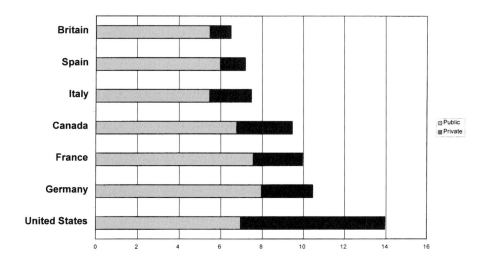

Figure 3.1.   Health Spending as %GDP 1997.

Decisions on the allocation of GDP to health are political. We have choices concerning the level of taxation that is acceptable; the priorities for private and State spending; and decisions on efficiency. On the latter point, it can be argued that the NHS is a very 'efficient' way to deliver health care, and there is much justice in this argument. However there is currently a growing consensus that health care in Britain is underfunded.

One possible explanation might be that expenditure on health has not been rising in real terms. However, as Figure 3.2 shows, the real cost of health has been rising year after year. The conclusion must be that Britain started from a low base and has not expanded the proportion of wealth dedicated to health care as the nation has become wealthier.

We must argue for two clear priorities. First, a greater proportion of national wealth to be spent on health and, second, for priority to be given to investment in primary care. Starfield (1994) shows that those health care systems with a robust, flourishing primary care system are more cost-effective.

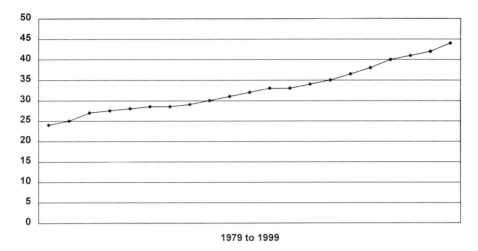

1979 to 1999

Figure 3.2. Health spending in the UK in real terms (£billion).

Workforce

The delivery of health care is a service. There are technologies but the essential element is the interaction between individuals. In order to deliver high-quality care, we need therefore sufficient high-quality staff in the health service. But what is 'sufficient'? Obviously the number of doctors will vary according to the configuration of the service. However a straight count of the numbers of doctors offers a gloomy picture of the British health system (Figure 3.3).

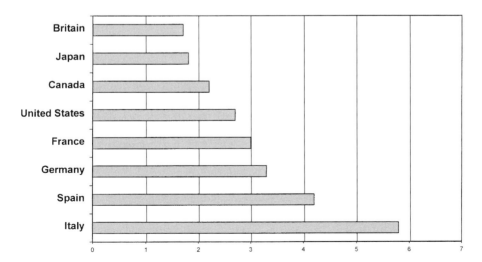

Figure 3.3. Doctors per 1000 population.

If a country chooses to deliver health care predominantly through doctors, then more doctors are needed to deliver the service. In Britain we have a much more team-based approach to care delivery, so there is a reasonable case for us to have fewer doctors. But we are not training enough doctors even for these deflated expectations. We are one of only two European Union countries that are net importers of doctors. We evidently need to train more doctors.

And how many general practitioners do we need? Inter-country comparisons are difficult. Italian general practitioners have average list sizes of just under 1000 patients. But Italian general practitioners usually have hospital or other appointments and work solo in general practice – without partners, nurses or receptionists.

When we look within the UK there is a better chance of a valid comparison. In England the average list size is 1850; in Scotland it is 1600. Geography or culture cannot explain this. It is an effect of a health service decision in Scotland to train sufficient doctors and to go for a quality service rather than for a 'make do and mend' service.

The only way that general practice has coped with expanding demand in recent years has been to expand the primary health care team. The practice in which I am a partner has been monitoring consultation rates for over 10 years. The rate has risen from just over four consultations per patient per year to nearly six. The rate of consultation with doctors has remained reasonably static at 3.5 per patient per year, because a greater number of nurse consultations has taken up the increase.

We therefore need to discuss the configuration of services that we wish to see and the skill mix that will be required to meet that configuration. For those of us who believe in the special clinical skills of doctors, there is a clear case for a reduction in list sizes, longer consultations with doctors and a sustained central role for general practitioners in the delivery of primary care.

Vocational training

When I completed my pre-registration house jobs I had a choice: go straight into general practice or undertake vocational training for general practice. During the course of my three-year vocational training scheme, vocational training became mandatory (in 1979). We were the first, and we remain the only, discipline in medicine to have our training detailed in legislation.

The training I undertook would be familiar to current general practice registrars. I did six months of psychiatry before entering my three-year rotation. I then had three months in my general practice; then four SHO posts in obstetrics, paediatrics, general medicine and 'specials'; and then nine months back in the practice. This was considered a remarkable opportunity in the 1970s and I took full advantage of it.

However, this model of training is beginning to break down. First, the idea that any trainer can appoint a registrar must be questioned. We must encourage young doctors who understand general practice and are suited to the discipline to enter vocational training. If we are to avoid a high attrition rate and prevent doctors unsuited to general practice from entering practice, we must select for training more rigorously.

The SHO posts must be reviewed. The service component overwhelms the teaching, and the teaching received is often poor and inappropriate. Many registrars do obstetrics, for example, just to get on the obstetric list and thus to earn higher fees. They then enter practice and do no intra-partum care. Is it really useful to have our future general practitioners doing six months of obstetrics, including a high commitment to the labour ward?

The demands of general practice have increased dramatically over the past 20 years. We have prevention, public health and health needs assessment, commissioning, financial management. . . . And the clinical agendum has increased enormously. It is no longer appropriate to consider one year in general practice as sufficient preparation.

The Royal College of General Practitioners, in conjunction with the General Practitioners Committee, is arguing for a voluntary extension of the general practice component of vocational training to 18 months. This should be available to all who wish it. Further, we believe that, if there is a consensus among the registrar, trainer and director that a further six months is educationally necessary, then this extension should be funded. This would make a maximum of two years in general practice.

Such a change would be dependent on a review of the content and training in the SHO posts and an improvement in the quality of hospital-based training.

We also recognise that there is a significant problem in the transitional period after vocational training. Many young general practitioners feel underprepared and choose periods as non-principals in order to become better equipped for general practice. We believe that there should be a voluntary system for higher training and mentoring which is called Higher Professional Training.

If these changes occur, we should be able to make general practice a more attractive career option, increase the quality of preparation for our discipline, improve morale, and enhance patient care.

The quality agenda

There is a wealth of activity in the area of quality, some directed by internal drivers and some in response to external events. The Shipman case has undoubtedly put us under the microscope in a way that is not necessarily comfortable. The General Medical Council's decision to introduce revalidation has created some remarkable challenges for us.

However, we must not forget that the quality agenda is our – the profession's – agenda. We have been working on quality programmes such a summative assessment, the MRCGP examination, Membership by Assessment of Performance, Fellowship by Assessment, and Quality Practice Award for years. We have espoused and supported clinical audit and are broadly supportive of clinical governance provided it remains professionally led.

One remarkable current change is the evolution from continuing medical education to continuing professional development. Ever since the publication of the CMO's report on continuing professional development (Department of Health 1998), we have been moving away from the 'bums on seats' idea of education towards an approach based on improvement in skills.

In continuing professional development, each doctor will be expected to reflect on the care they deliver and to identify strengths and weaknesses. Doctors will then address their weaknesses, resulting in an improvement in care. Let me illustrate.

I had a patient who came out of hospital after a myocardial infarction on a drug of which I'd never heard. I checked it briefly before prescribing it, but noted it for discussion. At the significant event meeting – we discuss every new coronary – I explained that I hadn't heard of this drug. One of my partners had and we agreed that I needed to update myself on anti-arrhythmic drugs. I looked in the British National Formulary and in Drugs and Therapeutics Bulletin. I found a recent editorial in a journal and I phoned a local cardiologist and checked my understanding. I then wrote a short protocol for the practice and we ran a computer search to see if any patients were on an inappropriate drug. We identified 14 such patients and marked their medical records. Subsequently I showed that some had been changed to more appropriate medication.

This is continuing professional development in action. I reflected on the content of the consultation with this man recovering from a myocardial infarction, and I then met my educational needs. I shared my new knowledge and applied it to improve patient care. I can almost guarantee that I would never have found a lecture to teach me what I needed to know. And I have learnt how to improve my expertise.

In the future I think it is inevitable that each of us will have a mentor with whom we have a regular appraisal. Such an appraisal will look at our standards of care, our continuing professional development, our career aspirations and how we can develop ourselves in a wider, professional sense. I would certainly welcome such an appraisal.

Around these quality activities, we have to put a mantle of regulation. It is not acceptable that there are some general practitioners delivering poor care – indeed possibly harming patients. We must reassure the public that every doctor is fit to practise.

We therefore need to offer a regular revalidation of all doctors, including all general practitioners. The Royal College of General Practitioners is working with other bodies, such as the General Practitioners Committee (RCGP 2000a), to design a system of revalidation for general practitioners. The standards used in revalidation will be based on those in *Good Medical Practice for General Practitioners* (RCGP 2000b). The process will be continuous, but with a regular – probably five-yearly – re-affirmation of registration.

If a general practitioner is found to be, or is thought to be, under-performing, a 'diagnosis' will be needed and appropriate support and help offered. We clearly cannot afford to lose significant numbers of doctors, so an assessment and support service will be needed to take a GP away from the practice, if necessary, and offer remedial help. For some doctors the problems will lie in health issues and we are arguing strongly for an occupational health service for general practitioners.

Access

The major political pressures and initiatives of the Blair Government have centred on the issue of access. Access to secondary care, as expressed through long waiting lists and delays in cancer treatment, is a high priority. However, a perceived poor access to primary care is also a major problem.

The invention of NHS Direct to offer faster triage and advice and of Walk-in Centres to offer faster consultation are two examples. These were introduced without a discussion about what improvements in access might occur if the same funding were applied to general practice itself.

It is of great concern when solutions to a perceived and acknowledged problem are developed without the involvement of those who know most about it – the general practitioners. However we are seen as part of the problem and have, as a profession, tolerated great variations in waiting time for appointments, poor telephone access and hurried consultations.

There is a real need for us as primary care professionals to define what access patients should expect. How long is it reasonable to wait for a routine, non-urgent appointment? How long should someone with an urgent problem wait? Should we offer some consultations out of office hours, in the evening or on Saturday? How can we argue for quality when some general practitioners are still offering five-minute appointments?

In particular we need to consider who should offer immediate care. For many practices, as discussed, nurses are doing more of the clinical care. Many nurses are now being trained to offer triage, to be the first point of contact for patients with urgent or new problems. This may offer a way to speed up access to assessment, deploying doctors for those patients that most need their medical skills.

Lastly, we need to be imaginative about out-of-hours care. General practitioner co-operatives are, by and large, a great driver for quality, but deputising services remains a source of considerable concern. We must ensure that good day time care with fast access is followed through into the night.

And this leads us full circle. If we are to offer better access to general practice, the simple truth is that we need more of it. We need more general practitioners, more practice nurses especially with higher training, more support and better premises. This country has to decide to address the fundamentals. Health service underfunding must be put right. The workforce needs to be expanded and nurtured. Primary care – the centre of the health service – must be developed.

References

Department of Health (1998). *A Review of Continuing Professional Development in General Practice. A Report by the Chief Medical Officer*. London: DoH.

RCGP and GPC (2000a). *Revalidation for Clinical General Practice. Draft Document for Consultation*. London: RCGP.

RCGP and GPC (2000b). *Good Medical Practice for General Practitioners. Draft Document for Consultation*. London: RCGP.

Starfield B (1994). Is primary care essential? *Lancet* **344**: 1129–1133.

▶ 4

Evidence-based General Practice

Yvonne H Carter, Maggie Falshaw, Sandra Eldridge

Development of evidence-based health care

The concept of evidence-based health care is not new but its development has accelerated over the past decade. Much of the impetus comes from within medicine and evidence-based medicine, or EBM as it has been commonly called, and it is an international phenomenon. In McMaster University in Canada David Sackett and colleagues developed EMB as a method of promoting life-long learning. More recently evidence-based health care has developed in a number of centres in the UK including the NHS Centre for Reviews and Dissemination at the University of York and the UK Cochrane Centre in Oxford.

Evidence-based health care has been described as 'the conscientious, explicit and judicious use of current best evidence in making decisions about the care of individual patients' (Sackett 1997). The practice of evidence-based medicine means integrating individual clinical expertise with the best available external clinical evidence from systematic research. This chapter will examine the development of evidence-based practice and its relationship to general practice and will consider the evidence from a recent trial conducted in primary care.

In its White Paper *The New NHS: Modern and Dependable* (Secretary of State for Health 1997) the Government stated that it would put quality at the heart of the NHS and it set out an ambitious and far reaching ten-year programme of modernisation, describing how the internal market would be replaced by a system of integrated care, based on partnership and driven by performance. The document promised early, visible improvements to the quality of service people experience in their own homes, at their GP surgery or health centre, and in hospital.

The White Paper focuses particularly on structures, quality and efficiency and six key principles underlie the changes set out:

▶ Renew the NHS as a genuinely national health service (set national standards).

▶ Devolve the responsibility for meeting these new standards to a local level (creation of primary care groups).

▶ Work in partnership (e.g. forging stronger links with local authorities).

▶ Improve efficiency so that all money is spent to maximise patient care.

▶ Shift the focus to quality of care ensuring excellence is guaranteed to all patients.

▶ Make the NHS more open and accountable to the public.

Under the new arrangements health authorities now take the lead in drawing up three-year health improvement programmes and have responsibility for improving overall health and reducing health inequalities. Following publication of *Our Healthier Nation* (Secretary of State for Health 1999), health authorities have a duty to improve the health of their population.

In *A First Class Service: Quality in the New NHS* (Secretary of State for Health 1998) the Government set out in some detail how it intended to implement the changes in England and it asked for views about how the objectives could best be met. The document emphasises the importance of the active participation of clinical professionals and patients throughout the NHS. The main elements of the proposals are:

▶ Clear national standards for services and treatments, through evidence-based national service frameworks and a new National Institute for Clinical Excellence.

▶ Local delivery of high-quality health care, through clinical governance underpinned by modernised professional self-regulation and extended life-long learning.

▶ Effective monitoring of progress through a new Commission of Health Improvement, a framework for assessing performance in the NHS and a new national survey of patient and user experience.

The establishment of primary care groups in 1999 has set a new agenda for service development and research in the NHS. *The New NHS* (Secretary of State for Health 1997), clinical effectiveness indicators and action on clinical audit place at the centre of the primary care agenda the delivery of health care that is research based, of proven efficacy and audited. All areas of the health service are being encouraged to develop a culture based on enquiry and the use of research evidence to inform practice. Evidence-based health care enables primary care workers to base decisions about diagnosis, treatment and management of patients on the best evidence available.

Using the best possible information to help in making clinical decisions is at the heart of evidence-based practice. Evidence-based health care and clinical governance aim to promote health care that is effective and that does more good than harm. This can only be achieved if relevant research findings and valid guidelines or recommendations are incorporated into practice. The research literature, however, varies in its degree of accuracy and completeness. For general practitioners to make properly informed decisions about care, it is essential that they have access to the best possible, most complete and up-to-date information they can find. Most people do not have the time to track down all the relevant research studies when trying to answer a clinical problem. Once the studies have been identified, it can also be both difficult and confusing to assess the quality and the sometimes conflicting results from different research studies.

Research findings can influence decisions at many levels: in planning care for individual patients, in the development of practice guidelines and in commissioning health care developing strategies for health promotion and preventive health. It can also be used in the development of policy both at a local practice, PCG, community trust and at a national level. But research findings can only play this role if research knowledge is translated into action.

Box 4.1. What is evidence-based medicine?

An approach to clinical problem solving

Areas: diagnosis, therapy, harm, prognosis

▶ Framing a question

▶ Searching for the best available evidence

▶ Appraising the evidence

▶ Making a clinical decision

In order to practise evidence-based care we need not only to have the evidence, but also to know how good the evidence is and whether it is appropriate for our patient populations. Traditionally most medical research, particularly using a randomised controlled trial design, has been based in hospital settings. There are differences between patients in hospital and the general population. If we take the example of patients with diabetes, those in the general population are likely to have fewer complications and their diabetes is likely to be better controlled than is the case with diabetes patients admitted to hospital. The diagnosis may be the same but there will be important differences in their health status. Because of these differences, research conducted solely with hospital patients will indicate different treatment regimens and thresholds than research whose subjects include patients at home.

The importance of primary care as a setting for clinical research has been recognised (Mant 1997, Medical Research Council 1997). Taken together these two reports published in 1997, the National Working Group on R&D in Primary Care chaired by Professor David Mant, and the Medical Research Council's Topic Review in Primary Health Care, have set the scene for a series of steps towards achieving the potential of an integrated clinical academic career structure in primary care. The Mant Report has been of relevance to all professional groups working in primary care and it set specific objectives including increasing the recruitment, development and retention of R&D leaders in primary care. In putting the case for supporting research and development in primary care, Mant explains that over 90% of contact between the population and the NHS takes place in primary care. Most minor illness is treated entirely in primary care and most serious disease presents first in primary care. In addition chronic illness is increasingly managed in primary care.

Primary care clinicians have responsibility in making decisions about diagnosis, referral to secondary care and prescribing medication. An evidence-based approach is important for all three. The need for a firm knowledge base is as important in primary as in secondary care. Much of the evidence required by primary care can only be obtained through research conducted in primary care settings that involves primary care practitioners and their patients.

Opportunities to engage in primary care research and development are growing and the scope for those wishing to become involved is finally widening. The Culyer Report (NHS R&D Task Force 1994) took steps to redress the underdevelopment of primary care research in relation to that in other sectors, by increasing the proportion of NHS R&D funding available for primary care. Infrastructure funding for research-active practices and the evolution of primary care research networks should both help to improve the research capacity and blur some of the boundaries between academic departments and clinical practice.

In 1999 the Central Research and Development Committee, which advises the Director of Research and Development at the Department of Health on the strategic framework and priorities for the use of the NHS R&D Levy, established a Strategic Review sub group, chaired by Professor Michael Clarke, to consider this framework. Five topic working groups were established in the following areas to facilitate this review: ageing, cancer, cardiovascular disease and stroke, mental health and primary care. The report on primary care (Clarke 1999) recommended that research needs to address the following areas: the demand for quality; the importance of partnership; the problem of inequality; and the generalist role and technological advances.

We are beginning to see an increase in primary care-based research, which is in turn leading to an increase in an evidence base for primary care decision-making. Translating research evidence into research practice will facilitate the promotion of effective health care. Lomas (1993) described three stages in the flow of research into practice: diffusion, dissemination and implementation.

How do GPs integrate the best available external clinical evidence with their individual clinical expertise?

Case study

A 63-year-old man attends morning surgery. He was discharged from hospital 2 months ago following a myocardial infarction. On examination his BP is 148/82, and his BMI is 27.2. He smokes 20 cigarettes a day. The results of a cholesterol test taken 12 months ago show his total cholesterol to be 6.1 mmol/l.

What sources of evidence would you use when planning how to reduce his risk of a further MI?

The man has several risk factors for heart disease:

▶ His age.

▶ Previous MI.

▶ Raised systolic blood pressure.

▶ His smoking status.

▶ Being male.

▶ His weight.

▶ His total serum cholesterol level.

Of these, changes could be made to his smoking status, blood pressure, serum cholesterol level and weight.

Evidence about the most effective way of achieving these changes can be obtained from a number of sources:

Box 4.2. Sources of evidence.

▶ Patient narrative

▶ Own experience

▶ Colleagues

▶ Experts

▶ Decision support: PRODIGY, Mentor, etc.

▶ Evidence-based databases

▶ Research papers

Patient narrative: a reduction in his risk factors is not achievable unless the patient himself is convinced and committed to making changes to his lifestyle. At this stage he may wish to discuss issues such as his concerns and anxieties following his myocardial infarction (MI). How will this affect his daily activities? Although many of these will have been discussed while he was in hospital he may want to talk about whether it is safe for him to drive and whether he can undertake strenuous activity. He may also have concerns about sexual activity or whether he will have a second MI. Such issues may need to be addressed before he feels able to discuss lifestyle changes to reduce his risk of a further coronary event.

His perspective is also important when looking at possible changes: any past experience of giving up smoking, his dietary preferences and beliefs, his attitude and fears about increasing his level of activity.

Patients' experiences, fears and health beliefs are an important source of evidence when planning risk reduction or other interventions.

Your own experience: although this is likely to be the start of your career in general practice, you are likely to have some experience of advising patients on risk factor modification. Experience about strategies and approaches that have or have not worked in the past are an important source of evidence. Any prior knowledge of the individual patient will also play a part. Consider which approaches are likely to work best with him.

Colleagues and experts are further sources of evidence. As a registrar your trainer has an important role in assisting your search for evidence for this patient. The vocational training scheme coordinator and other trainers may play a part. As a partner or non-principal your GP and practice nurse colleagues will also have useful advice and opinions for you to consider. The cardiologist responsible for inpatient treatment is another source. Local clinical guidelines on secondary prevention and risk factor modification may also have been produced.

Decision support software, such as PRODIGY and Mentor, is another important source of clinical evidence. Risk factor sources such as Framingham can be used to calculate the patient's absolute risk of a coronary event.

The growing number of evidence-based databases can be drawn upon.

Box 4.3.   Evidence-based websites.

Academic sites

University of Oxford: Health Services Research Unit

http://hsru.dphpc.ox.ac.uk/research.htm

Includes overviews of systematic reviews of effectiveness.

University of London: Institute of Education: Social Science Research Unit EPI Centre http://www.ioe.ac.uk/ssru/ra_epi.htm

The EPI Centre aims to promote evidence-based practice and practice-based research in health promotion and social interventions, to promote lay involvement in all stages of health research from setting the agenda to sharing and making use of the findings. The website provides a resumé of the work of the EPI Centre and a list of contacts. The list of current projects on the evaluation of interventions gives contact details.

Electronic journals

Bandolier: http://www.jr2.ox.ac.uk:80/Bandolier

Bandolier is produced monthly in Oxford for the NHS R&D Directorate. It contains bullet points (hence Bandolier) of evidence-based medicine.

Cochrane newsletter

http://www.update-software.com/ccweb/newslett/hpnews1.htm#Nuggets

UK Cochrane Centre health promotion newsletter.

Effective Health Care Bulletins

http://www.york.ac.uk/inst/crd/ehcb.htm

Effective Health Care is a bi-monthly bulletin for decision-makers which examines the effectiveness of a variety of health care interventions. EHC bulletins are produced by CRD and published by The Royal Society of Medicine Press Ltd.

Effectiveness Matters

http://www.york.ac.uk/inst/crd/em.htm

Effectiveness Matters is produced to complement Effective Health Care and provides updates on the effectiveness of important health interventions for practitioners and decision-makers in the NHS. It covers topics in a shorter and more journalistic style, summarising the results of high-quality systematic reviews.

Learning resources

CASP (Critical Appraisal Skills Programme)

http://www.his.ox.ac.uk/casp/

CASP is a UK project that aims to help health service decision makers develop skills in the critical appraisal of evidence about effectiveness, in order to promote the delivery of evidence-based health care. This website gives background information about CASP and provides contact details.

Other NHS and UK official sites

National Institute for Clinical Excellence – NICE (UK)

http:/www.nice.org.uk

NICE is a new Special Health Authority with a remit to appraise systematically health interventions before they are introduced in the Health Service. It offers clinicians and health professionals clear guidelines on which treatments work best for patients, and which do not. This website contains information about NICE, related news, links, FAQs and other information.

NHS Centre for Reviews and Dissemination, University of York

http:/www.york.ac.uk/inst/crd/welcome.htm

The NHS Centre for Reviews and Dissemination exists to provided the NHS with information on the effectiveness of treatments and the delivery and organisation of health care. Their Database of Abstracts of Reviews of Effectiveness (DARE) covers the published literature on effectiveness of health care interventions, while the NHS Economic Evaluation database concentrates on the economic aspects.

UK Cochrane Centre

http://www.update-software.com/ccweb/

Supports the NHS Research and Development Programme and is part of the worldwide Cochrane Collaboration.

Research papers: the increase in primary care research is reflected in the number of papers published in peer review journals.

Electronic databases are a useful tool for finding appropriate research papers. Medline is an international database of biomedical and associated health literature compiled by the National Library of Medicine in the United States. It contains references from approximately 3600 journals.

Medline can be accessed through the BMA website: www.bma.co.uk as well as through Medical School libraries. It can also be accessed through http://biomednet.com

Limitations of Medline

Although a Medline search is a useful place to start to look for references addressing clinical issues, it is not exhaustive. Medline covers 3600 journals but is geared towards American publications. A number of important journals such as *Health Service Journal*, *Health Education Journal*, *Quality in Health Care* and *New Scientist* are not listed on Medline.

Even when the references are on Medline you are not certain to pick them up. Sometimes the problems are caused by inadequacies in indexing. In general only 50% of the trials in Medline can be found by even the best electronic searchers. A study found that 18% of randomised controlled trials (RCTs) were found by experienced clinical searching; 52% with someone with optimal Medline searching skills; and 94% were found through hand searching (Sackett *et al* 1996).

Other researchers looked at identifying controlled trials published in the *BMJ* and *The Lancet* before and after a hand search of the literature. Only 21% of articles that could be found by hand were found through an electronic search (Jolly *et al* 1999).

The Cochrane Collaboration is working to overcome this information gap by hand-searching journals and incorporating any trials found into Medline. However, the Cochrane Collaboration can only work on a number of central areas and so much information will still be missed.

Although a Medline search will not be complete it is still likely to give references which are not relevant for your specific question. You will need to discard these. Some references can be discarded by looking at the title of the paper. However, you may still be left with irrelevant articles. Skim read the abstract of the articles to get an idea of which ones are worth keeping in your list and which you should discard. This is not foolproof. Abstracts are usually written to give a positive light to the article, but they can help you discard some articles which are inappropriate for your question.

The more experience you have of Medline searching the more skilful you become at it and your searches will be more complete and precise. Once you have found papers which may address the question, you need to read the papers and appraise their quality. You need to judge the research evidence.

The three main methodologies used in primary care research are: quantitative research, including RCTs and cohort studies; qualitative research and evaluation of cost effectiveness.

Critical appraisal of a therapy paper

In this appraisal we will focus on quantitative research and particularly the situation where two or more treatments, therapies or interventions are being compared as in a controlled trial, using the SHIP trial as a case study from general practice (Jolly *et al* 1999).

Box 4.4.

▶ What is the question?

▶ Were the patients randomly allocated to treatment groups?

▶ Were all the patients who entered the trial properly accounted for at the conclusion? Was follow-up complete? Were patients analysed in the groups to which they were allocated?

▶ Were the patients, health workers and study personnel 'blind' to the treatments?

▶ Were the patients in the groups treated equally?

▶ Were the patients in the groups similar at the start of the trial?

▶ How large was the treatment effect between the groups?

▶ How precise are the results?

▶ Can the results be applied to my patient care?

▶ Were all clinically important outcomes considered?

▶ Are the likely benefits worth the potential harms and costs?

In the SHIP trial practices not patients were randomised to intervention and control groups. This is not an uncommon practice in health services research, and is usually done when the intervention being evaluated is aimed at a practice level. Randomising individual patients in these circumstances could result in control patients being contaminated with the intervention if the practice to which they belong is receiving the intervention. These trials are often referred to as cluster randomised trials because clusters of individuals rather than single individuals are being randomised.

It will also be useful to read the associated editorial (Hobbs and Murray 1999), a second paper in the same edition of the *BMJ* on the development and evaluation of complex interventions in the SHIP study (Bradley *et al* 1999) and the correspondence that followed in the journal (Robson 1999, Mant 1999).

Before critically appraising the content of any paper you may want to look at the authorship and the references. This sets the paper in context. How many authors were there and what were their individual contributions to the project? Are they well known/known to you? How wide ranging are the references and, if you are familiar with the field, are the references what you would expect to see?

What is the research question?

To assess the effectiveness of a programme to coordinate and support follow-up care in general practice after a hospital diagnosis of myocardial infarction or angina? (706, Abstract: objective)

Were the patients randomly allocated to treatment groups?

In this study, the 'treatments' were interventions and these interventions were applied to practices not patients. Practices were randomly allocated (706, Abstract: design and

Participants and Methods: design). Details of how this was conducted and by whom are not given. It is not clear, for example, what is meant by 'practices were randomised before consent'. A previous paper is referred to as addressing details of recruitment and intervention (Jolly *et al* 1998), but does not contain much more information.

Were all the patients who entered the trial properly accounted for at the conclusion?

Yes (707, table 1). Of 597 patients who started the trial, 57 were lost to follow-up and 38 died, leaving 502 who were followed up at 1 year.

But what about practices? Initially 67 practices were recruited, 33 intervention and 34 control (706, Participants and Methods: design) but at least two (707, Participants and Methods: intervention) 'formally declined the participation of their practice nurses in the project'; three out of 33 intervention groups declined to take part (709, Discussion).

Was follow-up complete?

No. Ten percent of patients were lost to follow-up (707, Participants and Methods: study population, and table 1). However information for primary outcomes is not provided for all of those followed up at 1 year. The footnote to table 3 indicates that for most primary outcomes data are not available for between 5% and 6% of the 502 who were followed up.

If follow-up is not complete, as in this case, we have to consider what effect this might have on the results of the trial. If the results for those lost to follow-up or for whom data were not available could be included in the trial would this alter the conclusions? It is unlikely that adding the results for those lost to follow-up will increase the size of the difference between the intervention and control groups for primary outcomes; those lost to follow-up are likely to be less affected by the intervention. Results for the primary outcomes are not significant (Abstract, 706) and are likely to remain so with the addition of results from those lost to follow-up.

The 57 individuals lost to follow-up have been included in the analyses of the outcomes in table 4, under the assumption that they continued their baseline behaviour up to the 1 year follow-up date. This is likely to underestimate the intervention effect.

A formal analysis of the sensitivity of the results to assumptions made about the results of those lost to follow-up is called a sensitivity analysis, but none was carried out here.

Were patients analysed in the groups to which they were allocated?

Yes. Intention to treat analysis was carried out (708, Statistical Analysis). This type of analysis keeps individuals in the groups to which they were allocated for analysis purposes regardless of the group they end up in or of their adherence to protocol. It ensures that intervention groups remain balanced, by keeping individuals in their randomisation groups. Thus a fair comparison can still be made. There is some bias introduced in an intention to treat analysis but it is usually small (and smaller than the bias introduced by alternative procedures) and in the direction of underestimating the effect of the intervention.

Were the patients, health workers and study personnel 'blind' to the treatments?

Yes, as far as possible. Without blinding (preventing individuals knowing which arm of the trial study participants are in) there is a possibility that preconceived notions of some of those involved in the trial about the relative merits of the different interventions may affect results. In this study the individuals most likely to affect the results are the patients, and the nurses who carried out the clinical examinations at 1 year.

Patients could not be blind to the treatment they were receiving but whether they knew which arm of the trial they were in depends on what they were told when their consent was asked for. This is not clear from this paper, but a previous paper states that they were asked to consent to a 1 year follow-up. The implication is that they did not know, specifically, about the nature of the interventions, and thus were effectively blinded.

Health workers could not be blind, but the potential for bias in results is small. Study personnel (i.e. the nurse who did the clinical examination) had not been responsible for delivering the intervention to the patient (707, Design) but the authors state that 'we could not exclude the possibility of the nurse becoming aware during the examination of which group the patient's practice was in'. There is no indication of how many nurses became unblinded during this process, so the potential extent of any possible bias is unclear.

Apart from the experimental investigation, were the patients in the groups treated equally?

There is no evidence that patients were not treated equally.

Were the patients in the groups similar at the start of the trial?

There is imbalance in proportions with angina, % men and % smokers (tables 1 and 2). Results are reported separately for patients with angina and myocardial infarction in tables 3 to 5. They indicate some differences in the way that patients with the different diagnoses responded to the intervention. No allowance is made in any analyses for differences in the proportions of men and smokers. Possibly investigators felt that this imbalance was unlikely to affect outcomes.

We also need to consider whether practices in the two arms of the trial were similar at the start. No information is given about this.

How large was the treatment effect between the groups?

This question is asking both about the statistical significance of the results (have any differences between intervention and control groups arisen by chance or is there evidence that the intervention is actually associated with some change?) and the clinical importance (do the results have policy implications?).

For all primary outcome measures (table 3) 95% confidence intervals include zero. The results are therefore not significant. It is quite likely that any differences between control and intervention groups have arisen by chance.

E.g. total cholesterol 5.93 in control, 5.80 in intervention
Difference = –0.14 (not –0.13 probably due to rounding error)
95% CI: (–0.33,0.06)

This 95% confidence interval indicates a 95% certainty that if the intervention was applied to the population as a whole (no examination of what the population is yet – that comes later) then on average the cholesterol would be between 0.33 mmol/l lower than with no intervention and 0.06 mmol/l higher than with no intervention. Thus the study does not really indicate whether the intervention does harm or good, although on balance it looks as if there is a greater chance that it does good.

These results are consistent with there being no effect of the intervention, but they could also arise if there is an intervention effect that is too small to be picked up by this study.

The authors set out the sort of differences they felt were clinically important at the outset of the study: for example, a 0.35mmol/l difference in cholesterol, doubling of smoking cessation rates (707, study population). The study had a power of 90% or over to detect these. Thus, there was a 90% chance that the study would detect these sorts of differences if the intervention was capable of producing them. The difference found for cholesterol was –0.14, 95% CI: (–0.33 to 0.06), and the possibility that the intervention effects a lowering of cholesterol level by 0.33mmol/l, a value very near the marker set for clinical importance at the outset, cannot therefore be ruled out. While the result is not statistically significant it may be clinically important. The reported difference for smoking cessation is nowhere near the clinical importance marker set out at beginning of paper. However in the discussion (709) the authors state that 'the confidence intervals in table 3 indicate that we cannot exclude the possibility of small but clinically important reductions in total cholesterol concentration, blood pressure, and smoking'. If, as this suggests, a smaller change in smoking cessation is considered clinically important, this study was not powered to detect it.

How precise are the results?

The width of confidence intervals measures precision. This varies according to the outcome being considered.

Can the results be applied to my patient care?

The complex nature of the intervention means that here you need to consider not only whether the characteristics of your patients are going to be similar to those patients in the study, but also whether your practice and the wider organisational and structural framework in which it is set are similar to those that existed in the trial.

The study sample was drawn from the population of those admitted to hospital who had survived a first or subsequent myocardial infarction and all patients with angina of recent onset who had been seen in direct access chest pain clinic or admitted to hospital (707, Participants and Methods: design). Of such patients 723 were identified over an 18-month period; 686 patients judged well enough to participate in the trial were approached and 597 consented. We do not know anything about those who did not consent. Might the trial have had greater effect on them? Probably not. Only patients with new diagnoses were included, whereas other studies referred to in the introduction suggest that such interventions may have a greater effect on 'prevalent cases' (707, Introduction). The study was carried out in Southampton and SW Hampshire. Any organisational, structural and general practice features specific to this area may limit the transferability of results to other settings.

Were all clinically important outcomes considered?

Yes. The investigators considered a wide range of outcomes: primary risk factors, prescribing outcomes, use of health services, and symptom control and quality of life.

Are the likely benefits worth the potential harms and costs?

Probably not. This question is usually concerned with side-effects, and costs versus benefits. Side-effects are not relevant in this context. The benefits that the paper highlights are the increased attendance at rehabilitation sessions and follow-up visits to practice nurses. There was an 18% increase in attendance at rehabilitation sessions. Thus, for every 100 patients receiving intervention, 18 extra attended rehabilitation session. It appears necessary to treat 5.6 (100/18) patients to get one extra attending the rehabilitation session. This is a small return for the cost of the liaison nurse. On balance it does not appear that benefits are worth the costs.

This critical appraisal of a therapy paper deals with the extent to which the paper has clear aims and is focused (question 1), attempts to minimise and assess any potential bias (questions 2 to 6), and analyses and presents data in a way in which they can be clearly understood, interpreted, and assessed for usefulness in other settings (questions 7 to 11). Although the critical appraisal questions for other types of quantitative studies are different from those used here, the basic principles of trying to assess clarity, bias, interpretation and usefulness of results are the same.

With regard to the particular paper that we have appraised, this paper has a clear research question, and the investigators have attempted to minimise bias by using randomisation, blinding where possible, intention to treat analysis, and treating patients equally (aside from the experimental investigation) in the two arms of the trial. The losses to follow-up, and imbalance in the groups at baseline have been reported and some attempt has been made to deal with the effects of these. The analysis has been presented clearly. The findings of the study are largely negative although the clinical importance of some of the findings cannot be ruled out, and the precision of some results is not high. The usefulness of the results in other settings is more difficult to judge, given the complexities of the intervention being tested.

Some of the less desirable features of this trial/paper are the incompleteness of blinding, the lack of reporting about practice characteristics and non-consenting patients, the inability of the study to detect some clinically important outcomes due to inadequate power, and the uncertainty about transferability to other settings. At least two of these features, the incompleteness of blinding and the uncertainty about transferability are common features of health services intervention trials and a direct result of the nature of such interventions. The investigators also undertook a qualitative analysis (Bradley *et al* 1999) alongside the quantitative work, and this has allowed better judgement to be made about the transferability of the intervention to other settings. The qualitative work also helps to explain why the intervention may not have been as effective as the researchers had anticipated. Correspondence following the paper addressed the issue of the study's power (Robson 1999), suggesting that smaller differences than the authors had set as clinical importance markers could have been chosen, but this was counteracted by one of the authors (Mant 1999).

The trial may not have produced the results the investigators hoped for but the resulting paper still satisfies most of the criteria for a good therapy paper. As a result sound conclusions can be drawn from the results presented, which can be strengthened by the complementary qualitative work. The purpose of critically appraising a paper is to be able to make this sort of judgement about whether the results are generally sound and can be used as evidence on which to base medical practice. In this case the answer is yes.

References

Bradley F, Wiles R, Kinmonth AL, *et al* (1999). Development and evaluation of complex interventions in health services research: case study of the Southampton heart integrated care project (SHIP). *BMJ* **318**: 711–715.

Clarke M (1999). *NHS R+D Strategic Review Primary Care.* Leeds: Department of Health.

Hobbs R, Murray ET (1999). Specialist liaison nurses. *BMJ* **318**: 683–684.

Jolly K, Bradley F, *et al* (1998). Follow-up care in general practice of patients with myocardial infarction or angina pectoris; initial results of the SHIP trial. *Family Practice* **15**: 548–555.

Jolly K, Bradley F, Sharp S, *et al* (1999). Randomised controlled trial of follow up care in general practice of patients with myocardial infarction and angina: final results of the Southampton heart integrated care project (SHIP). *BMJ* **318**: 706–711.

Lomas J (1993). Diffusion, dissemination and implementation – who should do what. *Ann NY Acad Sci* **703**: 226–235.

Mant D (1997). *R&D in Primary Care: National Working Group Report.* Leeds: Department of Health.

Mant D (1999). Follow up care in general practice of patients with myocardial infarction and angina (Author's reply). *BMJ* **319**: 380.

Medical Research Council (1997). *MRC Topic Review: Primary Health Care 1997.* London: Medical Research Council.

National Health Service Research and Development Task Force (1994). *Supporting Research and Development in the NHS.* London: HMSO.

Robson J (1999). Follow up care in general practice of patients with myocardial infarction and angina (Letter). *BMJ* **319**: 380.

Sackett DL (1997). *Evidence-based Medicine; How to Teach and Practice EBM.* Edinburgh: Churchill Livingstone.

Sackett D, Rosenburg W, Gray J, *et al* (1996). Evidence based medicine: what and what it isn't. *BMJ* **289**: 587–590.

Secretary of State for Health (1997). *The New NHS: Modern and Dependable.* London: Department of Health.

Secretary of State for Health (1998). *A First Class Service: Quality in the New NHS.* London: Department of Health.

Secretary of State for Health (1999). *Our Healthier Nation.* London: HMSO.

Further reading

BMJ Publishing Group (1999). *Clinical Evidence. A Compendium of the Best Available Evidence for Effective Health Care.* London: BMJ Publishing Group.

Carter YH, Falshaw M (eds) (1998). *Evidence Based Primary Health Care. An Open Learning Programme.* Oxford: Radcliffe Medical Press.

Chambers R (1998). Clinical Effectiveness Made Easy: First Thoughts on Clinical Governance. Oxford: Radcliffe Medical Press.

Eldridge S, Ashby D (2000). *Master classes in research: Statistical concepts.* In: Carter YH, Shaw S, Thomas C (eds) London: Royal College of General Practitioners.

Thomas C (1996). Critical appraisal of the literature. In: Carter YH, Thomas C (eds). *Research Methods in Primary Care.* Oxford: Radcliffe Medical Press.

5

Audit – A Quality Tool in Health Care

John Schofield

Introduction

The problem with using audit as part of summative assessment is that it will for ever be viewed in a poor light just as a great novel studied for GCSE somehow loses its appeal.

I must admit to finding quality and audit fascinating. Used properly it allows one to improve the care that can be given to patients in a way that gets rid of the blame element endemic in medicine.

We are constantly bombarded by papers and protocols on how we could do better but are given very little support in long-term improvements. Audit is about doing things a bit better this month and a bit better the next and so on. It is a team effort with all the players having a say in how things are done.

I hope that you will be able to take a little from this and use it in your everyday practice. Just two points to emphasise before starting:

- Evolution rather than revolution.

- A no blame culture.

Getting started

Think first, then think again then have a cup of tea is my advice. Try to involve all the team at the start so that they feel that they have had a say in choosing a topic. Make it short, simple, understandable and relevant to the real problems that people experience. Most of all look at it from the patients' point of view and endeavour to make an early impact on the way that they view your service.

The theoretical ideal way of choosing a subject is to engage your community in questionnaires, focus groups and complaints analysis. I say community because you should address the problems of everyone not just the patients who are frequent surgery attenders.

One handy way round this is to use Pareto's principle which is that 80% of problems result from only 20% of the causes. In other words common things happen commonly. You can usually get a feel of what matters in a practice by asking everyone to note down when things go wrong. These can be plotted on a graph and should look something like the following (Figure 5.1).

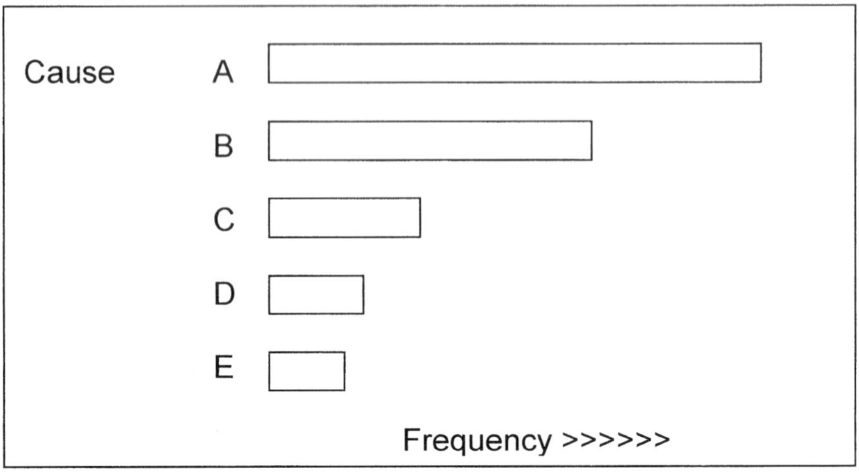

Figure 5.1. Pareto graph.

Having settled on a topic, you will find its worth looking up the literature to see if any other work relates to it. There are starting to be a number of websites that publish audits. Try EQUIP (below).

What type of audit?

You need to consider where best in the system to measure what you are doing.

Three types of audit are recognised:

▶ Structure – is a system in place?

▶ Process – are the procedures being followed?

▶ Outcome – are the outcomes satisfactory?

The great temptation is always to go for an outcome audit but this can be extremely difficult to achieve. There may be many factors that cause the result to vary and which are difficult to correct for. Practical experience shows that making sure that the structures and systems are in place and working effectively can have huge benefits with comparatively little effort.

Setting criteria and standards

This seems to get people. Criteria are measurable markers of how well you are providing a service. The standard is the level that you would hope to achieve for the

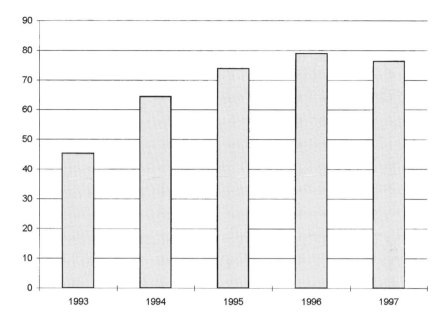

Figure 5.2. Audit of men aged 40–60 with blood pressure (BP) recorded on the computer.

criteria. To make it simple it is best just to take two or three criteria at most so that they can be easily recorded. A typical criterion might be 'Men between 40 and 60 years old should have their blood pressure recorded on the computer at least every 5 years' (Figure 5.2). It sounds very easy to do but I can assure you that it is not.

By the time we had achieved 80% it was actually starting to fall. Those that we had persuaded to come in at the start needed to be recalled.

By having access to this sort of material you can easily set a standard which is rather better than we achieved. Shall we say 85 or 90%? This is known as 'benchmarking'.

Collecting the data

Audit is very different from publishing a research paper in *The Lancet*. You are trying to get a feel for things. It is more akin to qualitative research. Having decided on a subject, set criteria that are meaningful and measurable, and find work to set your standards, for your next job is to sample the group in question. Try to do as little work as possible!

My favourite method of deciding on a sample size is gradually to increase the size of the sample (4, 8, 16 >>) until the result settles to a level. If you do this for the first time that you run the audit then, when repeating it, you can just use the same sample size. It should look something like (Figure 5.3):

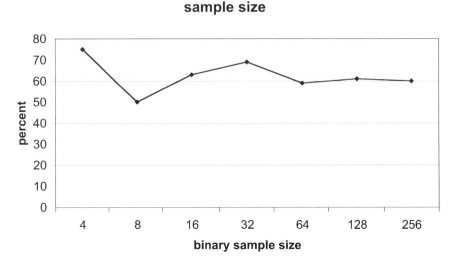

Figure 5.3. Deciding on your optimum sample size.

Making sense of data

So often work is presented in a huge confused table or as raw data that for the average person is impossible to follow. A clear description of what you were hoping to improve, how you decided on good markers of quality and what your findings were is a great art. Simple diagrams and graphs are always much more understandable than sheets of figures.

Having involved the team from the start, you need great tact when presenting the results as it can feel very threatening to see that you are not doing as well as you thought. Try above all to avoid blaming an individual but look instead to see if the system is at fault.

A flip chart to clarify everyone's role in the system is a great help. From this you can look at the systems and procedures that are in place and see if it is possible to improve them. Lots of little improvements can have a startling effect on the overall results. If you are a purist then flow charts, root cause charts and Pareto analysis help to clarify the situation. (I have not gone into these here but there are lots of books on the subjects and websites devoted to quality.)

Planning improvements

How about brainstorming the problem? Let everyone throw up ideas, jot them down on a flip chart and then tease out practical solutions. Write down what you are going to do in procedures, together with a date when you will rerun the audit. If possible steal someone else's good idea. It saves wearing your brain out.

Sharing your work

Tell everyone about your achievements: publish it on the Internet, write a newsletter for your practice, present your work at the postgraduate meeting. Be proud of what you have achieved.

Places where you can get help and ideas

There is a great deal of help out there. So do ask!

Local postgraduate centres can put you in touch with audit advisors for your local area. There are books on the subject and the government produces a great deal of material on quality improvement in the NHS. The *BMJ* runs the European Forum on Quality Improvement. Most of all the Internet is coming into its own. Here are a few websites worth visiting.

Box 5.1. Websites.	
EQUIP	www.equip.ac.uk
North Thames East GP Department	ntegpdep.tpmde.ac.uk
BMJ Quality	www.quality.bmjpg.com
Quality in the New NHS	www.open.gov.uk/doh/newnhs/quality.htm
Bandolier	www.ebando.com
National Centre for Clinical Audit	www.ncca.org.uk
National Library of Medicine (US)	lcgm.nim.nih.gov/

Box 5.2.   Books.
Measurement of Patients' Satisfaction with Their Care 　　Ray Fitzpatrick and Anthony Hopkins 　　Royal College of Physicians
Making Sense of Audit 　　Donald and Sally Irvine 　　Radcliffe Medical Press
Medical Audit in Health Care 　　Martin Lawrence and Theo Schofield 　　Oxford General Practice Series

Audit flow charts

Flow charts are used when possible in quality systems because they force one to be clear as to what is going to happen. One for doing an audit seemed appropriate at this stage (Figure 5.4).

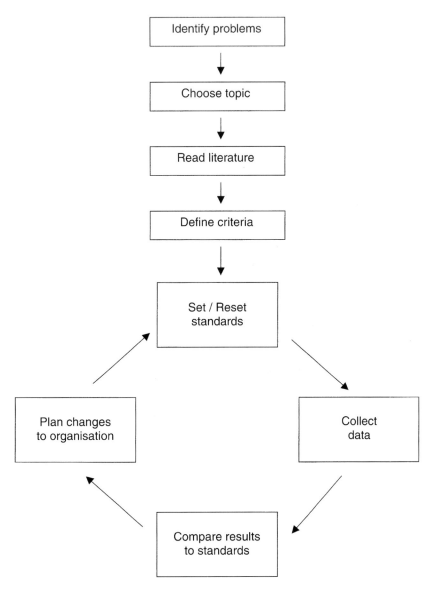

Figure 5.4. Audit Flow Chart.

Applying audit to quality improvement

An understanding of variability is what audit is about. The real world does not come in nice simple answers of yes and no. Everything is grey in varying shades and the harder you try to pin it down the more it slips away. Audit is merely a series of momentary snapshots of what is happening. What it does do is allow you to make best guesses of which direction to move.

Beside variability the other main features of Quality are Systems Thinking, Group Knowledge and the Motivation of the people. I am disturbed when audit is just taken on its own as the beginning and end of the solution to problems. It is not. Much more important is the motivation of people. They need to be involved in the decision process and then allowed get on with their job.

I am sure that you were all introduced to Gaussian distributions at college. These give a good picture of the real world. With quality what one is trying to do is to decrease the variability in a system and at the same time move to the top end of the spread so that everyone is assured of a good service.

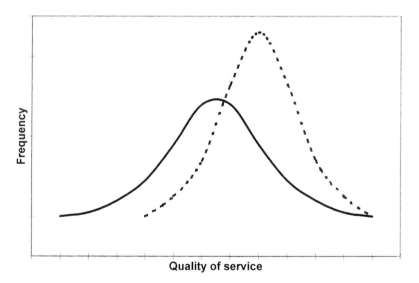

Figure 5.5. Quality of service. The solid line represents the present situation and the dotted one what one might hope to achieve in the future.

The end

Finally do not forget KISS (Keep It Short and Simple). May all your audits be little ones.

6

Prescribing

John Ferguson

Prescribing is a high-cost, high-profile activity and not likely to become less so in the future. Most GP consultations end with a prescription and English national prescribing statistics over the past 12 years show a steady upward growth of 4% in prescription items and nearly 10% in prescription costs over this period. Current figures (1999–2000) are 535 million prescription items at a cost of just over £5 billion, which is nearly 13% of the total cost of the NHS.

Prescription growth has undoubtedly occurred due to more care in the community by general practitioners over the years. A culture of care has been fostered in this country, with the belief that there is a pill for every ill. However, many prescriptions are still written for products which would be available over the counter for self-medication and it may be that our present system has fostered a dependent patient population. If we truly believed in patient empowerment, we should be encouraging patients to take responsibility for their own health and in the treatment of minor illness in the first instance. Our desire to appear helpful has perhaps fostered this dependent population who turn to their general practitioner in the first instance rather than trying a home remedy.

Currently over 80% of prescriptions are dispensed without charge and it has been estimated that approximately 50% of patients are exempt from prescription charges. However, these figures may change as a result of the recent counter-fraud activities. Prescription charges bring in about £350 million and so represent a very small fraction of the drug cost. But with increases in the prescription charge, we may now be coming to a point where those who pay prescription charges may feel that, if they need a simple remedy, it could be bought over the counter or obtained by private prescription more cheaply.

Have you ever thought what happens to all those prescriptions which you write and give to patients? The vast majority are dispensed and then these completed prescriptions are sent for independent pricing, payment of dispensing contractors and for information feedback to the NHS. In England this is done by the Prescription Pricing Authority which is a Special Health Authority within the NHS, but Scotland, Wales and Northern Ireland have their own pricing departments and issue their own prescribing reports.

A pilot computerised information system led to the development of a more informative and select information system called Prescribing Analysis and Cost (PACT). It was first implemented in August 1988 and an analysis of the scheme demonstrated that substantial savings in the drug budget could be achieved by using

PACT, by generic prescribing, therapeutic substitution and reducing inappropriate prescribing (Spenser and van Zwanenberg 1989). Within a year of the introduction of PACT the PPA showed that the number of high-spending doctors was decreasing, suggesting that feedback works.

Following the 1990 GP contract and the call for a more integrated approach to the rational effective use of medicines, it was clear the time had come for PACT reports to be updated and improved. Extensive consultations were undertaken with the profession and all those interested in prescribing information and, wherever possible, their suggestions were incorporated into the new PACT reports.

The PACT standard report (first issued in August 1994) is an eight-page A4 'landscape' report including a four-page article in the centre of the report. It is issued quarterly to all prescribers, health authority professional advisers, and appropriate sections of the NHS Executive and the Department of Health. The report is sequenced so that each page provides an increased level of detail. These are designed to be high quality, user-friendly reports with additional features such as the practice's top 20 drugs, generic prescribing and the proportion of new drugs included for the first time. Standard PACT reports contain, within a standard format, much individual practice-specific prescribing information. They are sent automatically to all GPs in England every three months towards the end of February, May, August and November. At the end of each quarter, in the course of ten working days, the PPA produces some 29,000 individual prescribing reports from its mainframe computer, through a high-speed laser printer.

The important features of these new PACT reports are now highlighted using a sample report (Figure 6.1) along with suggestions as to how the information can be used to monitor prescribing.

Page 1

Page 1 shows a simple bar chart of the practice's prescribing costs for the quarter compared with the Health Authority (HA) equivalent (average) and the national equivalent (average). The HA equivalent is based on the actual figures for the local HA adjusted to create an imaginary practice with the same proportion of patients aged 65 years and over. The national equivalent is created in the same way.

These equivalents allow practices to see how their prescribing compares with other practices in the HA or nationally. The individual GP's prescribing costs are also shown. Figures are given to show how these various costs have changed from the previous year.

Discussion point

If your practice's costs are above or below the local or national equivalent, you may want to find out why.

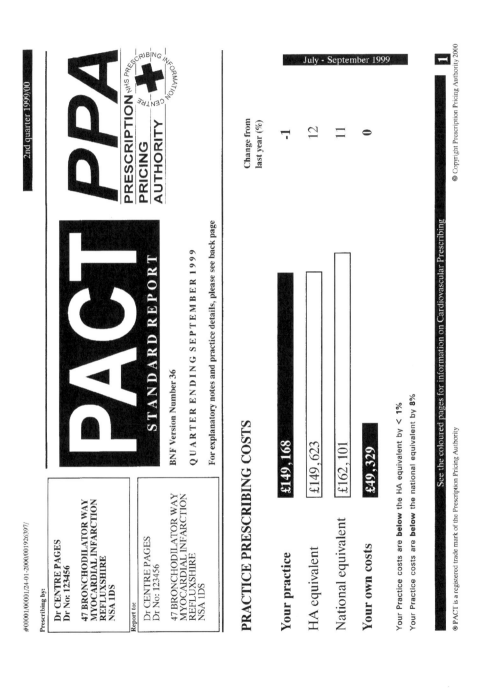

Figure 6.1. Sample PACT report.

YOUR PRACTICE COSTS BY BNF THERAPEUTIC GROUP

2 July - September 1999

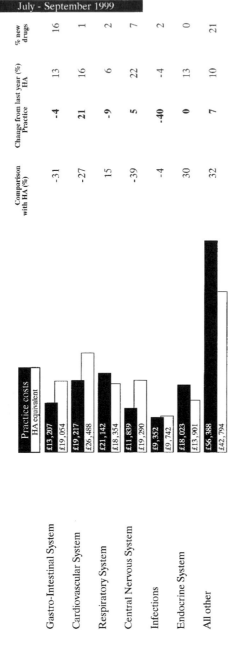

	Practice costs / HA equivalent	Comparison with HA (%)	Change from last year (%) Practice	HA	% new drugs
Gastro-Intestinal System	£13,207 / £19,054	-31	-4	13	16
Cardiovascular System	£19,217 / £26,488	-27	21	16	1
Respiratory System	£21,142 / £18,354	15	-9	6	2
Central Nervous System	£11,839 / £19,290	-39	5	22	7
Infections	£9,352 / £9,742	-4	-40	-4	2
Endocrine System	£18,023 / £13,901	30	0	13	0
All other	£56,388 / £42,794	32	7	10	21

THE TWENTY LEADING COST DRUGS IN YOUR PRACTICE

These drugs represent 37.6% of your total practice cost. G: generic form available

Drug	Total cost (£)	% practice total	Change from last year (%)	No of items
1: Genotropin	9,150	6.1	-3	21
2: Omeprazole	6,025	4.0	53	159
3: Havrix	5,076	3.4	55	250
4: Becotide G	2,982	2.0	-44	129
5: Augmentin	2,981	2.0	-7	356
6: Typbim Vi	2,745	1.8	-24	257
7: Becodisks	2,549	1.7	-9	53
8: Eprex	2,543	1.7	99	6
9: Beclometh Diprop (Inh)	2,498	1.7	15,057	155
10: Ranitidine HCl	2,277	1.5	170	78

Drug	Total cost (£)	% practice total	Change from last year (%)	No of items
11: Adalat G	2,190	1.5	17	83
12: Fluvirin	2,138	1.4	0	420
13: Proprietary Co Enteral Nutrit	1,877	1.3	1	34
14: Influenza (Mericux)	1,867	1.3	-	366
15: Mengivac	1,786	1.2	39	267
16: Amoxycillin	1,758	1.2	303	1,833
17: Recormon	1,580	1.1	-25	2
18: Cyclosporin (Systemic)	1,475	1.0	5	6
19: Amlodipine Besyl	1,272	0.9	-9	42
20: Ins Humulin I (Isop)	1,248	0.8	38	24

THE NUMBER OF ITEMS YOUR PRACTICE PRESCRIBES

		Change from last year (%)	Prescribed generically (%)	Dispensed generically (%)
Your practice	23,083	-4	45	43
HA equivalent	16,532	2	58	52
National equivalent	19,478	3	57	52
Your own prescribing	7,229	-2	42	40

The number of items your Practice prescribed is **above** the HA equivalent by **40%**
The number of items your Practice prescribed is **above** the national equivalent by **19%**

PRESCRIBING BY BNF THERAPEUTIC GROUP IN YOUR PRACTICE

July - September 1999   3

	No. of items prescribed	HA equivalent	Comparison with HA (%)	Change from last year (%) Practice	HA	Dispensed generically (%)
Gastro-Intestinal System	1,413	1,207	17	**15**	7	25
Cardiovascular System	1,253	2,709	-54	**22**	9	51
Respiratory System	4,078	1,553	163	**-17**	-3	36
Central Nervous System	3,055	2,688	14	**-6**	4	55
Infections	3,104	2,048	52	**-22**	-11	80
Endocrine System	996	1,067	-7	**2**	8	55
All other	9,184	5,260	75	**7**	5	30

AVERAGE COST PER ITEM

		Change from last year (%)
Your practice	£6.46	3
HA equivalent	£9.05	9
National equivalent	£8.32	7
Your own average cost	£6.82	2

The average cost of items prescribed by your Practice is **below** the HA equivalent by **29%**

The average cost of items prescribed by your Practice is **below** the national equivalent by **22%**

THE AVERAGE COST BY BNF THERAPEUTIC GROUP IN YOUR PRACTICE

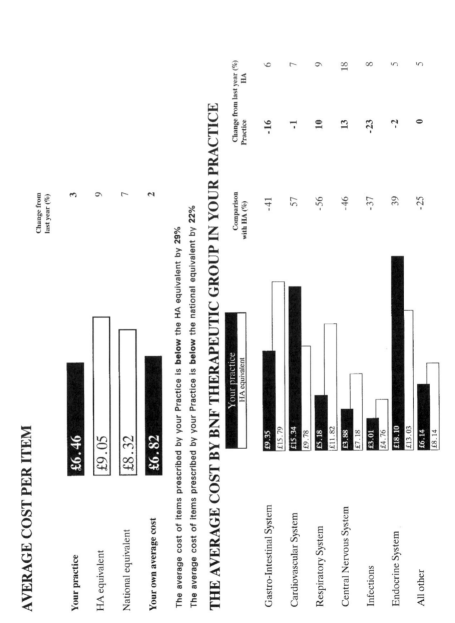

Your practice / HA equivalent

		Comparison with HA (%)	Change from last year (%) Practice	HA
Gastro-Intestinal System	£9.35 / £15.79	-41	-16	6
Cardiovascular System	£15.34 / £9.78	57	-1	7
Respiratory System	£5.18 / £11.82	-56	10	9
Central Nervous System	£3.88 / £7.18	-46	13	18
Infections	£3.01 / £4.76	-37	-23	8
Endocrine System	£18.10 / £13.03	39	-2	5
All other	£6.14 / £8.14	-25	0	5

CORONARY HEART DISEASE PRESCRIBING

Trends in Cardiovascular Prescribing in England (Chart 1)

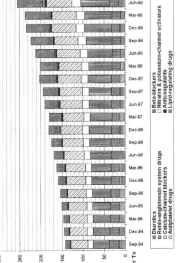

Trends in Cardiovascular Spending in England (Chart 2)

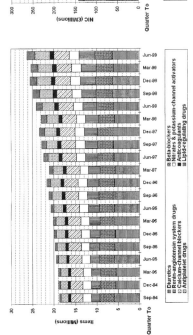

Coronary Heart Disease (CHD) is a major cause of death accounting for about a quarter of all deaths under the age of 65. Circulatory diseases are estimated to cost the NHS and the personal social services some £3.8 billion annually. They account for 35 million working days lost each year and cost industry more than £3 billion a year. Saving Lives: Our Healthier Nation contains a target to reduce the death rate from CHD and stroke related disease in people under 75 years by at least two fifths by 2010, saving up to 200,000 lives in total.

The forthcoming National Service Framework on Coronary Heart Disease reflects the importance placed by the government on tackling this problem.

The burden of CHD is not distributed equally in society. For example, men of working age in the lowest socio-economic class are 50% more likely to die from CHD than men in the population as a whole. There is also a geographical variation with people living in the North of the country more likely to die from CHD compared with the South.

Over the last couple of years there have been several new guidelines on the management of cardiovascular disease, including the Joint British recommendations on the prevention of coronary heart disease in clinical practice (Heart 1998; 80: S1–S29) and the British Hypertension Society (BHS) guidelines for hypertension management (summary in BMJ 1999; 319: 630–635).

The approach of both of these guidelines is to assess risk factors and then use drug therapy where indicated, targeting those at highest risk first. All cardiovascular risk factors should be looked at rather than focusing on a single risk factor and treating it in isolation.

CHD is associated with a combination of factors, some such as age, sex and family history of heart disease are unalterable whilst other factors related to lifestyle are modifiable and can be influenced. These include hypertension, hyperlipidaemia, diabetes mellitus, smoking, obesity and lack of physical exercise.

Hypertension, hyperlipidaemia and diabetes mellitus are associated with a particularly high CHD risk. The new guidelines recommend a target blood pressure of 140/85 mmHg or lower and total cholesterol less than 5.0mmol/L and LDL cholesterol less than 3.0mmol/L. For patients with diabetes mellitus the BHS guidelines recommend a target BP of 140/80 mmHg.

Smoking is estimated to be associated with 18% of CHD deaths. Passive smoking may increase CHD relative risk by 25%. The cardiovascular benefits of stopping smoking are apparent within 1 year in all age groups. A recent MeReC bulletin discussed nicotine replacement therapy concluding that it is an effective intervention for smoking cessation. Nicotine replacement products are not generally available on the NHS; however, limited supplies may be available in Health Action Zones.

Obesity increases the risk of CHD by increasing blood cholesterol and BP. A 5kg weight loss in patients who are greater than 10% overweight reduces BP by 5 mmHg in a significant number of individuals. A diet including plenty of fruit, vegetables, fibre, oily fish and low in saturated fat and salt will assist in the reduction of cardiovascular disease.

Physical inactivity doubles the risk of CHD. Modest aerobic exercise helps prevent hypertension and myocardial infarction. Whilst moderate alcohol consumption reduces CHD risk, this message needs careful communication to patients reminding them to remain within the advised limits.

It is no surprise that Cardiovascular is the top BNF chapter in terms of both number of prescriptions and cost. For the quarter to June 1999, 22% of all prescriptions (28 million) were for cardiovascular drugs. Cardiovascular prescribing accounted for 22% of the spending for this quarter (£276 million).

Over the last 5 years the number of prescriptions for all the main classes of cardiovascular drugs has increased (Chart 1). Diuretics have increased by 13%, beta-blockers by 17%, whilst lipid-regulating drugs have shown a 350% increase.

Chart 2 shows an overall increase in spending over the last 5 years. Antiplatelet drugs, lipid-regulating drugs and anticoagulants have shown the largest increases, over 5 fold for antiplatelet and lipid-regulating drugs and over 9 fold for anticoagulants.

The following table shows the place of the major cardiovascular drug groups as a percentage of total prescribing and spending on cardiovascular drugs for the quarter to June 1999. These major groups account for 93% of all prescriptions for cardiovascular prescribing and 92% of spending.

	Items	Cost
Diuretics (BNF 2.2)	22%	6%
Beta-blockers (BNF 2.4)	14%	8%
Renin-angiotensin system drugs (BNF 2.5.5)	13%	24%
Nitrates & potassium-channel activators (BNF 2.6.1/2.6.3)	8%	8%
Calcium-channel blockers (BNF 2.6.2)	13%	21%
Anticoagulants (BNF 2.8.1/2.8.2)	3%	2%
Antiplatelet drugs (BNF 2.9)	13%	2%
Lipid-regulating drugs (BNF 2.12)	7%	22%

Diuretics - thiazide diuretics remain one of the first line drug choices for treating hypertension They now account for 40% of diuretic prescriptions (2.5 million per quarter) but only 15% of spending on diuretics (£2.3 million). Bendrofluazide (bendroflumethiazide) is the most commonly prescribed thiazide at 92% of thiazide prescriptions but 63% of spending. Over the last 5 years there has been a therapeutically rational move towards prescribing the 2.5mg in preference to the 5mg tablet. Prescriptions for loop diuretics are 33% (2.1 million) at a cost of 36% (£5.8 million) of all diuretics. The use of potassium-sparing combination diuretics has fallen over the last 5 years but they still account for 22% of prescriptions (1.4 million) and 43% of the spending or £6.8 million per quarter.

The prescribing of spironolactone has fallen over the last 5 years. The Randomized Aldosterone Evaluation Study (RALES - N Engl J Med 1999; 341: 709-17), looking at 1663 patients with severe heart failure, showed that the addition of 25mg of spironolactone to conventional treatment (ACE inhibitor, loop diuretic and in most cases digoxin) significantly lowered risk of all-cause mortality, death from progressive heart failure and sudden death. At this low dose of spironolactone, serious hyperkalaemia or azotaemia were rare. In the light of this study spironolactone prescribing may increase.

Beta-blockers - atenolol remains the most commonly prescribed beta-blocker at 60% of prescriptions (2.4 million per quarter) and 32% of costs (£6.8 million). Propranolol is the second most commonly prescribed, 15% of prescriptions and 12% of costs. Bisoprolol accounts for 5% of prescribing and 14% of the spending.

Drugs affecting the renin-angiotensin system - the number of prescriptions for ACE inhibitors has increased by more than 70% over the last 5 years and is currently over 3 million prescriptions per quarter at a cost of £56 million. Lisinopril and enalapril are the most frequently prescribed ACE inhibitors at 34% and 28%. Audits have found that ACE inhibitors are under-used for heart failure but frequently prescribed for patients with hypertension where no contraindications for the use of thiazides or beta-blockers exist.

Since their introduction the use of angiotensin-II receptor antagonists has increased steadily and they now account for 418,000 prescriptions (£11.4 million) per quarter. The BNF reminds us that angiotensin-II receptor antagonists are a useful alternative for patients who have to discontinue ACE inhibitor therapy because of persistent cough but beyond this their role in the management of hypertension remains to be established.

Nitrates and potassium-channel activators - isosorbide mononitrate remains the most commonly prescribed nitrate at 59% of prescriptions (1.2 million per quarter) and 77% of costs (£14.2 million). Prescribing of the more expensive isosorbide mononitrate modified release preparations has increased (59% items, 91% costs). Glyceryl trinitrate is the second most commonly prescribed nitrate, 36% of prescriptions and 21% of costs. Since its introduction nearly five years ago, the use of nicorandil has increased steadily and it now accounts for 160,000 prescriptions (£2.5 million) per quarter.

Calcium-channel blockers are not a homogeneous group having disparate therapeutic effects. Prescribing of this group has increased by 32% over the last 5 years and is now 3.6 million prescriptions per quarter at a cost of £59.3 million. Over the last 5 years there has been a marked shift in prescribing from standard preparations taken several times a day towards once daily longer acting preparations.

Anticoagulants - warfarin is highly effective at preventing strokes in patients with atrial fibrillation. The prescribing of warfarin and low molecular weight heparins has increased over the last 5 years. Prescriptions for warfarin have almost doubled to 889,000 per quarter whilst spending has increased to £3.4 million. Currently low molecular weight heparins account for 0.7% of prescribing (5,900 items per quarter) and 15% of spending (£610,000) in this group.

Antiplatelet drugs - low-dose aspirin is by far the most commonly prescribed antiplatelet at 95% of prescriptions (£3.4 million per quarter). As can be seen from the cost chart aspirin 75mg dispersible tablets are inexpensive and aspirin only accounts for 52% of the spending on antiplatelet drugs. The place of aspirin in secondary prevention of all atherosclerotic vascular disease is well established. For primary prevention the BHS guidelines recommend 75mg of aspirin for hypertensive patients aged 50 years or older who have satisfactory control of their BP (less than 150/90 mmHg) and either target organ damage or diabetes or a 10 year CHD risk equal to or greater than 15%. Clopidogrel prescribing has increased rapidly since its introduction a year ago and although it is only 0.5% of prescriptions in this group this amounts to 16% of the spending. Dipyridamole accounts for 4% of prescriptions and 28% of the costs.

Statins - there is strong evidence from clinical trials to support the prescribing of statins to reduce LDL cholesterol in patients at high absolute risk of CHD. However, to make the best use of resources these drugs have to be targeted at those patients with the highest risk. Details of appropriate tables or risk calculator computer programmes to use are included in the recent guidelines. Two years ago there was a four fold difference between health authorities in spending on statins (NIC per 1,000 lipid lowering STAR(97)-PUs) This variation is now less and there is currently a two and a half fold variation. Statins now account for 88% of lipid-regulating prescriptions (1.7 million items) and 92% of the spending (£57 million per quarter). Simvastatin remains the most commonly prescribed statin at just over half of all prescriptions.

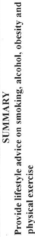

<table>
<tr><td>
SUMMARY

- Provide lifestyle advice on smoking, alcohol, obesity and physical exercise
- Determine all risk factors and use these to estimate 10 year CHD risk
- Aim to reduce BP to 140/85 mmHg or lower
- Actively manage hypertension using thiazides and beta-blockers as first line drugs where appropriate
- Low dose aspirin is effective and cheap
- Target statins to patients at highest risk of CHD
- Use ACE inhibitors in heart failure rather than in hypertension
</td></tr>
</table>

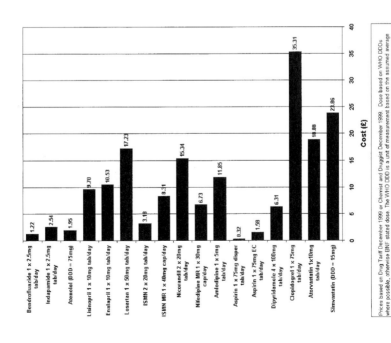

Cost For 28 Days Treatment

Drug	Cost (£)
Bendrofluazide 1 x 2.5mg tab/day	1.22
Indapamide 1 x 2.5mg tab/day	2.54
Atenolol (DDD = 75mg)	1.95
Lisinopril 1 x 10mg tab/day	9.70
Enalapril 1 x 10mg tab/day	10.53
Losartan 1 x 50mg tab/day	17.23
ISMN 2 x 20mg tab/day	3.18
ISMN MR 1 x 40mg cap/day	8.31
Nicorandil 2 x 20mg tab/day	15.34
Nifedipine MR 1 x 30mg cap/day	6.73
Amlodipine 1 x 5mg tab/day	11.85
Aspirin 1 x 75mg disper tab/day	0.32
Aspirin 1 x 75mg EC tab/day	1.58
Dipyridamole 4 x 100mg tab/day	6.31
Clopidogrel 1 x 75mg tab/day	35.31
Atorvastatin 1x10mg tab/day	18.88
Simvastatin (DDD = 15mg)	23.86

Prices based on Drug Tariff December 1999 or Chemist and Druggist December 1999. Dose based on WHO DDDs where possible, otherwise BNF stated dose. The WHO DDD is a unit of measurement based on the assumed average maintenance dose in adults. It may not necessarily reflect the actual dose used.

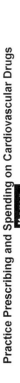

Practice Prescribing and Spending on Cardiovascular Drugs

Snr Partner:Dr CENTRE PAGES
47 BRONCHODILATOR WAY

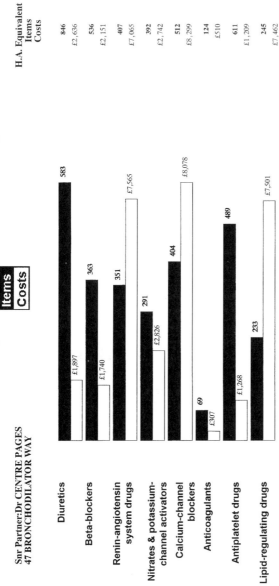

		H.A. Equivalent Items Costs
Diuretics	583	846 £2,636
	£1,897	
Beta-blockers	363	536 £2,151
	£1,740	
Renin-angiotensin system drugs	351 £7,565	407 £7,065
Nitrates & potassium-channel activators	291 £2,826	392 £2,742
Calcium-channel blockers	404 £8,078	512 £8,299
Anticoagulants	69 £307	124 £510
Antiplatelet drugs	489 £1,268	611 £1,209
Lipid-regulating drugs	233 £7,501	245 £7,462

	Practice		H.A. Equivalent	
	Items/1000 PUs	Cost/1000 PUs	Items/1000 PUs	Cost/1000 PUs
ACE inhibitors	46.51	972.67	52.84	879.26
Angiotensin-II receptor antagonists	4.50	127.05	4.28	112.43
Nicorandil	3.34	79.95	2.67	42.71
Aspirin (antiplatelet)	63.96	81.55	78.37	64.97
Statins	30.96	1,023.98	29.85	967.97

YOUR TOTAL PRACTICE PRESCRIBING COSTS BY BNF THERAPEUTIC GROUP FOR THE PAST TWO YEARS

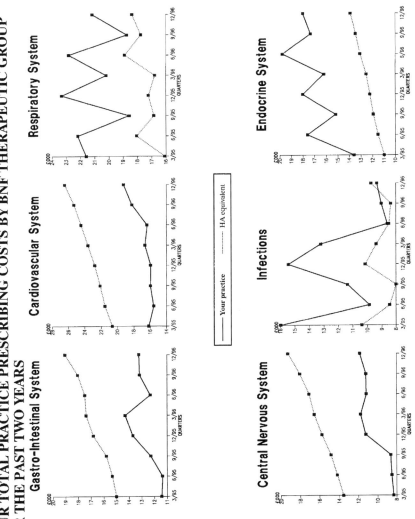

YOUR PRACTICE'S TOP 40 BNF SECTIONS BY COST
Items and costs by section

6 | July - September 1999

Ranking			Costs £	Compared with HA (%)	Compared with Last year (%)	Items No	Compared with HA (%)	Compared with Last year (%)
36	1.1	Antacids	838	22	30	364	64	33
3	1.3	Ulcer-Healing Drugs	9,744	-30	-7	286	-29	0
29	1.6	Laxatives	1,122	-29	26	304	-14	13
21	2.4	Beta-Adrenoceptor Blocking Drugs	2,254	-24	-6	260	-44	26
7	2.5	Antihypertensive Therapy	7,372	-21	22	270	-39	33
6	2.6	Nit,Calc Blockers & Potassium Activators	7,592	-4	35	384	-31	22
26	2.12	Lipid-Lowering Drugs	1,238	-69	40	32	-73	45
9	3.1	Bronchodilators	5,780	-12	-11	1,016	31	-22
2	3.2	Corticosteroids	10,101	4	-8	394	-8	0
13	3.4	Allergic Disorders	3,421	317	-3	1,153	616	-13
31	3.10	Systemic Nasal Decongestants	963	999	-18	667	1,158	-13
23	4.2	Drugs Used In Psychoses & Rel.Disorders	1,440	16	37	55	-62	-10
12	4.3	Antidepressant Drugs	4,428	-46	35	281	-50	27
38	4.6	Drugs Used In Nausea And Vertigo	765	-13	-43	135	-19	-16
14	4.7	Analgesics	3,047	-35	-12	2,239	118	-11
39	4.8	Antiepileptics	741	-61	23	84	-55	14
33	4.9	Drugs Used In Park'ism/Related Disorders	852	-36	-11	44	-51	-14
5	5.1	Antibacterial Drugs	8,422	10	-41	3,015	57	-22
10	6.1	Drugs Used In Diabetes	5,256	16	28	554	54	6
16	6.4	Sex Hormones	2,836	-51	0	148	-49	3

4	6.5	Hypothalamic&Pituitary Hormones&Antioest	9,463	299	-11	39	225	-24
32	7.3	Contraceptives	885	-52	-12	223	-38	-3
34	7.4	Drugs For Genito-Urinary Disorders	846	-9	94	41	-16	41
18	8.2	Drugs Affecting The Immune Response	2,395	61	27	26	30	44
30	8.3	Sex Hormones & Antag In Malig Disease	1,025	-61	47	10	-82	-37
11	9.1	Anaemias + Other Blood Disorders	5,217	456	16	743	427	8
17	9.4	Oral Nutrition	2,712	2	28	69	-30	97
24	9.6	Vitamins	1,401	322	-31	312	243	-18
8	10.1	Drugs Used In Rheumatic Diseases & Gout	6,691	9	-23	970	37	4
19	10.3	Drugs For Relief Of Soft-Tissue Inflamm	2,270	152	8	437	191	15
35	11.4	Corti'roids & Other Anti-Inflamm.Preps.	842	328	-18	132	187	-1
28	12.2	Drugs Acting On The Nose	1,191	8	-7	169	8	-27
22	13.2	Emollient & Barrier Preparations	1,513	14	2	459	52	12
15	13.4	Topical Corticosteroids	2,981	108	1	795	78	0
37	13.5	Preparations For Eczema And Psoriasis	796	-16	-19	54	17	-17
25	13.6	Preparations For Acne	1,324	52	41	153	125	17
20	13.10	Anti-Infective Skin Preparations	2,261	102	24	497	131	17
1	14.4	Vaccines And Antisera	13,864	106	34	1,630	67	41
27	19.2	Selective Preparations	1,203	824	9	911	3,861	15
40	20.3	Wound Management & other Dressings	686	-68	-10	47	-67	-8

8 | July - September 1999

PRACTICE PROFILE

	Total list size	Patients 65 & over	Temporary residents	No. PUs
Dr CENTRE PAGES	3,565	230	35	4,025
Practice	9,343	534	105	10,411

TOTAL PRESCRIBING ASCRIBED TO YOU

	Items	Cost (£)
Dr CENTRE PAGES	7,229	49,329
Trainee	-	-
Community Nurse (P) for the practice	-	-
Deputising services for the Practice	1	9

ITEMS PERSONALLY ADMINISTERED OR DISPENSED BY YOUR PRACTICE

	Personally Administered		Dispensed	
	This year	Last year	This year	Last year
Practice cost	£8,221	£7,493	n/a	n/a
- of total practice cost	5.51%	4.98%	n/a	n/a
No. of items	1,505	1,175	n/a	n/a
Av. cost/item	£5.46	£6.38	n/a	n/a

Overall av. cost/item £6.46   Last years overall av. cost/item £6.28

EXPLANATORY NOTES Please refer to the PACT/IPS Technical Guide for more detailed explanations.

HA Equivalent Throughout this report all figures represented as "HA equivalent" are based on the actual figures for the local HA adjusted to create an imaginary practice with the same number of PU's as your practice.

National Equivalent Throughout this report all figures represented as "National equivalent" are based on the actual figures for England adjusted to create an imaginary practice with the same number of PU's as this practice.

Change from Last Year The % change from the equivalent period last year.

Costs Total Net Ingredient Cost.

Therapeutic Groups The six therapeutic groups listed are those which incurred the highest costs in England from April 1999 to March 2000.
The term "All other" includes preparations, dressings and appliances.

New Drugs For the purposes of PACT, drugs are classified as new for a period of three years after the receipt by the PPA of the first prescription for a black triangle drug (CSM monitored).

Leading Cost Drugs These drugs using names by which they were prescribed, are those which contributed the most to your costs. All presentations are added together to obtain the figure for each drug. Drugs you have prescribed using a proprietary name and for which a generic form is available, are identified by the letter **G**.

Dispensed Generically % figures for items prescribed by the approved name, even when a generic is not available (excludes dressings, appliances and adjuncts).

Total List Size The total number of patients registered with the practice (including temporary residents and over 65s) as last notified by your HA.

Temporary Residents The list size shown for temporary residents is based on the same quarter of the previous year and is included in the total list size.

Prescribing Units (PU) Patients under 65 years of age and temporary residents count as one PU Patients aged 65 or over count as three.

Trainee These figures represent all prescribing on your prescription forms that have been marked with a "D" in red ink.

Community Nurse (P) These figures represent all prescribing on FP10(PN) prescription forms by qualified community practice nurses who are part of your practice team.

Deputising Services These figures represent all prescribing by deputising doctors who have used prescription pads stamped with "L" and specified the senior partner number of your practice.

Personally Administered Items prescribed and administered by you or a member of your practice team and which attract payments under para 44.5 of the Statement of Fees and Allowances (Red Book).

Dispensed Items dispensed by a dispensing practice including any personally administered items.

% figures for items where a generic is available and the dispenser has been paid for a generic (excludes dressings, appliances and adjuncts).

You are now able to request full details of your prescribing in the form of a prescribing catalogue.

For more information contact: Help Desk, Prescription Pricing Authority, Block B, Scottish Life House, Archbold Terrace, Jesmond, Newcastle-upon-Tyne, NE2 1DB, Tel:(0191)2035050 Fax:(0191)2035001

Page 2

On page 2 the practice prescribing costs (and HA equivalents) are broken down into the national top six British National Formulary (BNF) therapeutic areas: currently, in order, gastro-intestinal, cardiovascular, respiratory, central nervous system, infections, endocrine, and other. Alongside the costs in each therapeutic area is a figure giving the percentage of prescribing costs in each area that is due to new drugs. Drugs are defined as new for three years after their introduction. (Only new drugs that carry the Committee on Safety of Medicine's (CSM) special surveillance (black triangle) symbol are included.)

Also on this page is a list of the 20 leading cost drugs in the practice giving the number of prescriptions, their total cost, the percentage of the practice total and the change from last year. In addition, brand-name drugs in the list are flagged with a 'G' if a generic preparation is available.

Discussion points

▶ The bar chart on page 2 can indicate therapeutic areas where costs are different from the local equivalent. Are there any reasons for these differences?

▶ The top 20 leading-cost drugs highlight individual drugs that are costing the practice a lot of money. Is the prescribing of these drugs appropriate?

▶ Where branded products in this list are marked with a 'G' it may be worth finding out how much may be saved by switching to the generic.

Page 3

This page concentrates on the number of items prescribed rather than costs. An item is equivalent to each order for a product written on a prescription form, but the amount prescribed is not considered. The chart shows:

▶ The number of items prescribed by the practice compared with HA and national equivalents;

▶ The percentage of items written generically;

▶ The percentage actually dispensed generically.

Discussion points

▶ How does your practice compare with the HA and national equivalent?

▶ What is the difference between the generic prescribing percentage and the dispensed-generically percentage (for dispensing practices)?

▶ Does the practice have a policy on generic prescribing?

Page 4

Page 4 combines the elements of the earlier data to provide details of the average cost per item for the practice compared with the HA and national equivalents. The average costs per item are also shown in each of the therapeutic areas.

Discussion point

The average cost per item will depend largely on the amount prescribed on each prescription and may well reflect practice policy on repeat prescribing. If costs per item vary widely from the averages you may want to find out why.

Page 5

Six graphs on page 5 show the changes in practice prescribing costs and HA equivalents over the last eight quarters in the six main therapeutic areas, demonstrating seasonal variation.

Discussion points

▶ Seasonal variation.

▶ How prescribing policy changes affect costs, e.g. increased use of anti-inflammatories in asthma.

▶ Whether the practice spending is converging or diverging from local patterns of prescribing.

Pages 6 and 7

An extensive table on pages 6 and 7 ranks the practice's own top 40 sections of the BNF in terms of cost. The number of items prescribed in each section is given along with comparisons with the HA and the practice's last year figures.

This table allows the practice to identify the therapeutic sections that account for the largest proportion of its spending on drugs. These may be the sections that the practice may wish to concentrate its attention on through the use of the more detailed information available in the prescribing catalogue.

Discussion point

Is prescribing in the most expensive therapeutic areas rational?

Page 8

Practice details such as list size are carried on the back page together with details of items personally administered or dispensed by the practice. If these details are not approximately correct, then the comparative percentages calculated throughout the report will not be correct. These items are those that attract payment under paragraph 44.5 of the Statement of Fees and Allowances (Red Book). A glossary of terms is also included on this page.

PACT centre pages

There is an insert in the centre of the standard PACT report that is concerned with some important and topical aspects of prescribing in general practice. It is illustrated by national trends in prescribing and looks at the quality issues raised by this aspect of prescribing. There is additional practice-specific prescribing feedback related to the topic of the centre page. The topics, which are published on a quarterly basis, have so far covered: asthma and inhalers; diuretics and potassium therapy; depression and antidepressants; hormone replacement therapy; antibiotics; lipid lowering drugs; analgesics and NSAIDs; contraceptives; wound management; cardiovascular drugs; respiratory drugs; ulcer healing; diabetic drugs; dermatological drugs; epilepsy; lipid lowering drugs; asthma prescribing; antibiotics, gastro-intestinal prescribing, diabetes and cardiovascular prescribing. The editor of this section is the Medical Director of the Prescription Pricing Authority, and there is also a multidisciplinary editorial board. The intention is primarily educational.

These new PACT reports have been well received and have generated much spontaneous comment. The editor of the Drug and Therapeutics Bulletin thought 'new PACT had impact'. The *British Medical Journal* editorial believed that the 'new PACT reports make the best prescribing data in the world even better'. A GP simply thought it was 'PACT with information'.

The prescribing catalogue

Prescribing catalogues are available only on request. These reports provide details of every item prescribed and dispensed by the practice or individual GP. As a result the full report runs to about 100 pages. A prescribing catalogue may be requested for the practice overall, or for individual partners or registrars, or if so desired it may be restricted to one or more individual therapeutic areas.

The first few pages of the report repeat information provided in the standard report and give additional details of prescribing rates. The remainder sets out in detail every item that has been dispensed in the quarter, with the quantity prescribed and the cost. It also sums the total number of tablets/doses prescribed per presentation. The catalogue flags products available generically (GFA), new drugs (N), controlled drugs (CD), CSM monitored drugs (CSM) and borderline substances (BS) – foods, alcoholic beverages and toilet preparations.

The prescribing catalogue and audit

The prescribing catalogue is by far the more valuable of the two reports if a practice wants to look in detail at its prescribing patterns or to monitor the effects of any changes in prescribing policy. The sheer volume of information provided may be daunting, but the key to success is to tackle it in manageable stages.

Limitations of PACT

PACT data are valuable but, as with any statistical information, they have their limitations and potential pitfalls. GPs need to be aware of these in order to avoid drawing the wrong conclusions and using the data inappropriately. It does not identify individual patients, any clinical factors or repeat prescribing.

Comparisons with HA and national equivalents

The population characteristics of an individual practice are unique and may vary enormously within one HA. Prescribing in any practice is determined in part by the characteristics of the patient population. When comparing prescribing with local and national averages demographic factors need to be borne in mind, as PACT data are not very sensitive to them.

Prescribing units

PACT data recognise that elderly patients generally require more prescriptions than patients in other age groups. Thus, for comparative purposes, the patient population in England is described in terms of prescribing units, or PUs. Under this system, patients of 65 and over count as three PUs on the crude basis that they require on average three times as many prescriptions as the under 65s.

The bar charts in the standard PACT report compare each practice with a fictional average or equivalent practice. The figures for this average practice are obtained by dividing the total costs or total number of items in the HA in that quarter by the total number of PUs in the HA. This gives an average cost or number of items per PU in the HA. These figures are then multiplied by the number of PUs in your practice to give the costs and number of items for a practice of similar size and age profile prescribing at the average rate for the HA.

ASTRO-PUs

The Prescribing Support Unit in Leeds has developed a weighting system: the age, sex and temporary resident originated prescribing unit (ASTRO-PU) that takes greater account of the differing prescribing needs of males and females in nine different age bands. It allows more accurate comparisons between practices and is already being used to help calculate prescribing budgets.

Practice list size

The prescribing and cost rates given in PACT are based on the practice list size held by the HA. While this is fine in areas where the population is stable, prescribing and cost rates may not be accurate where the list size is rapidly changing. Data for individual partners are also based on their personal list size; unless GPs see only patients registered with them, and use only their own prescription forms, individual comparisons with practice and other equivalents are of little value.

Cost per item

When looking at cost per item for the practice compared with HA and national averages it is important to remember that this figure depends on the quantity of drug prescribed each time. A practice that always issues repeat prescriptions for three months will have a higher cost per item than a practice that prescribes one month's treatment. Cost per item should be looked at in conjunction with the quantity prescribed.

Individual GP prescribing

PACT data for individual GPs relate to the prescriptions written on the GP's prescription pad or under that doctor's unique prescriber number. Where one doctor's FP10s are used for repeat prescribing or nurse-requested items or where the GP registrar uses the trainer's pad, the PACT data are distorted. For audit purposes aggregated practice data should be requested.

Electronic PACT (EPACT)

Professional prescribing advisers need to be able to cope with a vast amount of PACT data for their health authority, and so an electronic Management Services Information System (MSIS) has been developed for them along with the PACTLINE analysis package that was first released in 1992. This provides electronic prescribing information on a monthly basis down to BNF chapter and section level. Prescribing patterns and trends can be readily identified and easily understood graphs and reports can be produced.

EPACT is the next step in the development of further prescribing information that was started by PACTLINE. It was produced by the PPA to enable professional advisers to obtain prescribing information down to individual drugs, and was implemented in a phased manner between November 1994 and March 1995 to all 100 HAs in England. Because of the size of the database, it was impossible to download this information, so EPACT was developed as a 'client/server' application to allow HA advisers to gain access to prescribing information held on the PPA's mainframe computer. Queries are generated by the individual adviser and may be requested for any number of practices or subsets over a range of time. Trends in drug use are identified by asking the same question on a monthly basis.

PACT and the future

Prescribing is an important activity in general practice. The majority of consultations end with a prescription. The Government's new White Papers on Health integrate individual general practices into primary care groups (PCGs) to provide a locally responsive National Health Service. The prescribing information needs of these PCGs will be different and we are planning to introduce new prescribing reports to meet this need. We are currently introducing an electronic PACT system running on the NHS net to provide this information.

The aim at the PPA is to collect and feed back more information electronically. With the advances in personal computers and networks, we can envisage the time when the GP will prescribe on his computer, send the prescription electronically to the pharmacist and then on to the PPA for pricing and reimbursement and prompt information feedback.

Quality prescribing will lead to effective health care. Use of statins for example has increased exponentially since the publication of the 4S study and the WOSCOPS report and now account for over £62 million per quarter. There is considerable variation between the 100 health authorities in England in the usage of statins. There is little correlation between the coronary heart disease mortality rates and the usage of statins, some areas having high statin usage and low mortality rates whilst others have low statin usage with high mortality rates. Overall usage is highest in the north west of England where mortality rates are medium to high. Statin usage is lowest in the West Midlands where coronary heart disease mortality rates are also high. The general trend in the South of England is of higher rates of statin usage than would be expected by the coronary mortality figures. So more needs to be done to target the use of statins to those at greater risk.

This government is determined to use information technology to improve the health care of patients. Electronic prescribing and data linkage will improve the quality of prescribing and we at the PPA are keen to play our part in this revolution.

All the recent changes in the NHS are designed to ensure quality standards of prescribing across the country. National Service Frameworks and NICE will issue guidance, CHI will monitor them and PCGs and PCTs will have to develop protocols of care for common general practice conditions. Though much of this guidance comes from the top, there will have to be ownership at a local level for it to be effective. Only in this way will a consistent level of care be provided with appropriate prescribing. As

Aneurin Bevan said in 1948 at the inception of the NHS, the aim is to 'universalise the best'.

Reference

Spenser JA, van Zwanenberg TD (1989). Prescribing research: PACT to the future (editorial). J R Coll G P **39**: 270–272.

► 7

Commissioning and Health Systems

Peter Orton

Primary care developments over the past 10 years have been an evolutionary process towards managed care. The White Paper on Primary Care published in 1997 (DoH 1997) accelerated the pace of change and led to the current development of the commissioning model of managed primary care.

Western health care systems are going through a time of rapid change and these changes will affect all those involved in providing health care. Health systems are facing pressure to spend more as demands for health care services increase. In the UK over the past 10 years GP consultations have increased by 15% and new attendances at casualty departments have increased by 20% (Secretary of State for Health 1999). As a result the principle of managed care is being established to contain costs. As managed care develops so health care professionals will become more accountable for their use of limited resources. In addition in the UK, health care expenditure is significantly lower than the level of national income would suggest, on the basis of other countries' expenditures. The pressure on resources appears to be greater in the UK than that experienced by other OECD countries (Judge and New 1996).

The principles of commissioning mean that all general practitioners are commissioners of health care, working together with other general practitioners on a locality basis. The process involves a commissioning cycle where the medical problem and thus the specific health need of the local population is identified before the services are purchased. A strategic approach to the problem is taken that influences the contract specification. An evaluation of health gain is made afterwards and this influences the need assessment for the next commissioning cycle. Health care is now based on the three 'Es' of evidence, effectiveness and efficiency, with a clear shift from quantity to quality of care. The focus now is on a local community approach, quality of care and the integration of management in the purchasing and provision of health care. Commissioning is not new and has been around for the past 10 years. It has evolved from both fundholding and non-fundholding models. Fundholding has evolved through multifunds and total purchasing pilots (TPPs), with non-fundholding evolving through GP forums and non-fundholding groups towards the commissioning model. In 1996 fundholding involved 3000 funds and 38% of general practitioners (3735 practices) covering 19 million people. The commissioning model had 84 funds and 24% of general practitioners (2800 practices) covering 14.3 million people. Previous fundholders have had clear advantages over non-fundholders when commissioning became the work of primary care groups. Fundholders have previously had a disproportionate share of health resources and had many of the skills required for commissioning in place. These include skills such as management, budgeting, prioritisation of resources and experience in handling the contract process.

In 1997 the White Paper on the NHS for England, *The New NHS*, was published with subsequent papers for Scotland and Wales. Its principles were that the NHS should be professionally led by primary care; the purchaser–provider split should remain, but responsibility should be decentralised; there should be national standards of care with an evidence-based approach, increased accountability, and the unification of the general practice (GMS) and community (HCHS) budgets. Above all health inequality should be reduced. Fundholding became extinct in 1999 with commissioning being the only model. The current commissioning model has four levels of involvement with increasing accountability and responsibility for the commissioning groups, as the levels evolve from just advising the Health Authority to becoming a Community Trust.

An average commissioning group (PCG) covers a population of 100 000 people with groups of 50 general practitioners working together with the local Health Authority. The Health Authority provides some of the management resources, remains responsible for some of the specialist care and provides other skills such as public health. Of particular interest is that commissioning groups now include the district nurses – which has and will mean a fundamental change in their role and working practice. The working together of a large number of general practitioners will cause problems for both team working and decision-making, but it will provide many benefits. The traditional hierarchical structure of practices, with doctors in control, now contrasts greatly with the task-orientated structure of the new commissioning groups. Mission statements implemented by a strategic and operational team now drive the commissioning groups. This change in structure will alter the balance between doctors, nurses and managers. The evolution of commissioning groups (PCGs) has meant some significant differences from the earlier models of managed care. These are: compulsory GP membership, collective responsibility, strategic planning, power sharing with other professional groups, an executive management and the move towards a unified budget. In theory the current influence of patient demand on the use of resources will be reduced and replaced by the clinical needs of the local population. One of the main principles of the White Paper was to reduce health inequality. With fundholding there was widespread inequality of health services with a two-tier health system. While commissioning may remove the previous inequality for some health services, this may now be replaced with some health services not being provided at all.

For the first time the allocation of resources for primary health care are based on a health needs formula rather than the historical use of health resources. It has been estimated that this redistribution of resources will produce winners and losers (Bloor and Maynard 1995). Losers would include the South West (−14%), London (−5%) and East Anglia (−7%). Winners would include Northern (+10%) and West Midlands (+7%). This level of redistribution of health resources, if achieved, will have a large impact with a difficult transition phase.

With fundholding there were few penalties. Funds that incurred debts were written off and the debts did not accrue from year to year. This had a corresponding effect on the funds available for non-fundholders. In addition any fundholding savings were kept by the fund. It is not clear what happened to the fundholding surpluses and debts but it is clear that what happened previously with the fundholding funds will not be allowed to continue. Commissioning groups now have a fixed budget, which is likely to be reasonably generous in the first two years. But as funding becomes more restricted commissioning groups will face difficult decisions in the prioritisation of the use of resources if the budget is overspent. The result will be some form of rationing and it is the commissioning groups functioning at the higher levels (Primary Care Trusts), where there is increased accountability and responsibility, that are most likely to run into problems with budget deficits.

Health Improvement Programmes (HIMP)

There are a number of issues currently facing primary health care. There still exist within the UK wide differences in health between different areas of the country. Some of the difference relates to social factors but another important reason is the variation in the performance of health professionals. The quality of medical care varies regionally, within communities and within practices. The changes in primary health care over the past 10 years have created a limited market but have largely focused on quantitative measures of outcome.

The use of qualitative outcomes of health has been uncommon. Despite initiatives to audit clinician behaviour and to implement changes in the doctor's behaviour there has been little change. The process of changing care involves assessing the problem, implementing changes and auditing performance. Change in clinical behaviour is more likely if management is involved in the process, working in conjunction with the medical profession. Previously the medical profession has tended to work separately.

An example within general practice of the wide variation in clinical behaviour is the prescribing of the antibiotic group cephalosporins.

Antibiotic prescribing is only one example of many areas in clinical medicine with there is a wide variation in clinical behaviour. An audit of all NHS prescriptions for the last quarter of 1996 by Health Authorities (Figure 7.1) showed a six-fold variation in prescriptions for cephalosporins. This variation in doctor-prescribing behaviour is unlikely to be explained purely on the basis of variation of the antibiotic sensitivities of the bacterial pathogens and the prevalence of bacterial injections. Clearly there are patient and doctor behavioural factors. With the current concern with drug costs and antibiotic resistance there are important implications.

One of the main concepts of the recent primary health care changes is the focus on quality of care, based on the health of a local community. Rather than individual practices and individual patient's needs being met, the health needs of the local community are becoming the focus. Local health needs will be set as targets, which will be monitored and compared with agreed national and local health criteria and

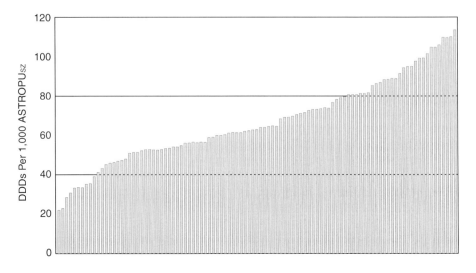

Figure 7.1.   Health Authority usage of cephalosporins (1996 – 4th Quarter).

standards. The new primary care groups (PCGs) consist of groups that reflect the local community such as: social services, patient representatives, public health officers and pharmacists.

In the first year the process of quality of care monitoring has been set up and those health problems identified which are relatively easy to assess. The current national topics are coronary heart disease and stroke, accidents, cancer and mental health. National guidance on some of these medical topics have and are being developed. Local communities, through their Primary Care Groups, are in many cases adopting two of the national topics in the first year.

An example of the process is seen within a local Primary Care Group. Within each of the four areas the problems relating to the local community have been identified. In coronary heart disease and stroke the locality has a standardised mortality rate (SMR) of 93, which is higher than other local communities, and so has been identified as a target area. Within accidents the SMR for road traffic accidents is high at 167, in cancer the SMR for melanoma is high at 149 and mental health depression in the elderly has been identified as a particular problem for the local community. From these four specific problems two have been taken forward for the first year; these are CHD and depression in the elderly. In future years non-medical topics are likely to be chosen that involve other care agencies that will require greater team-working. The process of implementation will have to be carefully planned and will involve both management and the medical profession in a new working relationship. It is likely that the balance between the two professional groups will shift with less autonomy for the medical profession.

Example: CHD

Taking as an example, the prevention of further cardiac events in post-myocardial infarction cases, the issues can be explored further. Current knowledge shows that in this group of patients, aspirin can prevent further major cardiac events; 25 patients need to be treated with aspirin for 1 year in order to prevent one myocardial infarction or death (NNT 25). A recent audit of these patients in a practice showed that two in three patients were on aspirin within the last year, out of some 60 cases that had had a myocardial infarction. Thus, provided that there were no contraindications to taking aspirin, one additional myocardial infarction or death could be prevented each year in this practice.

This example shows how audit can be applied to the quality of care using an evidence-based approach. The process involves non-medical groups, such as educational material by the local general practitioner education group and the use of a trained audit facilitator aiding the audit process within the practice.

However there are a number of problems with the Health Improvement Programme. Resources are already scarce and the funding of PCGs will be different from the previous allocation of funds. The process has been largely based on historical patterns. For the first time a resource allocation working party (RAWP) formula will be applied to general practice, such as has previously only been applied to secondary care. This will be seen as the PCG national formula and will result in a reduction in funding for some areas (South and Southwest) and an increase in other areas (North). New skills in audit, needs assessment and people management will require a training programme. Accurate and timely information will be required on which to measure performance and to plan. Much of this information is often incomplete or late and, with the loss of fundholding activity analysis, practices will need to develop accurate data collecting methods. Current health authority data on general practice is often incomplete and inaccurate.

Perhaps the greatest challenge is changing behaviour. There has been very little change in behaviour with the Health of the Nation initiative. Clearly with a shift in focus towards the quality of care, measuring change will become more important in determining outcomes. To change behaviour involves both a stick and a carrot approach. It is currently unclear as to what the balance will be and whether the medical profession's local medical committees will take on the policing and monitoring role. If the profession itself does not take on this role then management certainly will with the resultant reduction in the autonomy of the profession. Overall the current changes in the health system offer some exciting possibilities in the move from quantity to quality of care. There is, however, a real danger that quality could be sacrificed as the standard of care moves towards a Mini rather than that of Rolls-Royce.

Summary

Quality of care has now become central to the changes now taking place in health care with the development of national guidelines, based on clinical excellence for primary care. In secondary care, quality is being developed through clinical governance and the implementation of quality standards in the contracting process. However, the effect of guidelines is likely to be the reduction of clinical freedom due to the move towards their being 'only one way to skin a cat'. As the range of acceptable clinical behaviour is reduced so flexibility of clinician behaviour will also be affected.

The White Paper on health for Scotland and Wales had some fundamental differences. Commissioning groups do not exist but instead there are primary health care trusts or local health groups. These include all primary health care and many of the services currently covered by community trusts. i.e. mental health.

With the proposed changes managed care is evolving further with management taking a much stronger role. The new primary care groups have many similarities with the health maintenance organisations (HMSO) of the USA. These primary care groups could equally well function in a private health care system.

The proposed changes for UK health care include many positive aspects but there are some serious concerns. Doctors are likely to become increasingly accountable and responsible for the provision of health services and the use of resources. At the same time doctors will see a reduction in their autonomy and clinical freedom. While UK health care remains underfunded, compared to many other Western countries, the proposed changes mean that the provision of care will be restricted; difficult choices will have to be made as to the level of health need to be met. Health care rationing is real.

References

Bloor K, Maynard A (1995). Equity in primary care. University of York, Centre for Health Economics Discussion Paper 141: October.

DoH (1997). *The New NHS*, White Paper. London: HMSO.

Judge K, New B (1996). UK health and health care in an international context. Health Care UK 1995/96, Kings Fund.

Secretary of State for Health (1999). Departmental Report. Department of Health: HMSO.

▶8

Practice Management

Eleanor Brown

In looking at the topic of practice management, both for your immediate needs in passing your exam and for practical use in the future, I would suggest covering the following areas:

- ▶ The history of practice management.
- ▶ Future functions and structure of primary care.
- ▶ Requirements of practice management in 'The New NHS'.

History of practice management

It is sometimes easier to look for characters in entertainment to help us understand the development of practice management. The obvious character which comes to mind for the first type of manager is that of Janet from Dr Findlay's Casebook. You may well be too young to remember this, but Janet was the live-in housekeeper to Dr Cameron, who was the true old-fashioned doctor living in the Scottish village of Tannochbrae, who had an answer or cure for everyone. A lot of his insight came from the information which Janet gave him. She was the person who kept him organised and managed his life, whilst he got on with looking after the patients. In close succession there was Dr Findlay's wife (Dr Findlay succeeded Dr Cameron as Senior Partner) who not only took over from Janet in organising the background support to the doctor, but also answered calls made by patients, judged their priority for visiting, and also seemed to have a dual role of instructing the sick on how to get better. There was definitely an element of 'triage' involved. Again, someone organised the doctor's life so he could get on with looking after the patients.

Still in this series of 'Dr Findlay' there was Mistress Niven who was the district nurse and midwife, but undertook a vast amount of work to support the doctor. All these three roles were very supportive and very subservient to the doctor, who was all-seeing, all-knowing and all-everything.

The real change in the tasks which were required, other than supporting and managing the daily routine of the doctor, i.e. cooking meals, organising patient appointments and answering the telephone, came about during the 1960s; the whole payment system to general practice took on a far more positive view with the change in GMS remuneration associated with the beginning of the 'health centre' approach. Suddenly, there was a revolution in the numbers of people working in primary care and an ability of the GP to be reimbursed for people who worked with a general practitioner. This was closely followed by monies which could be made available to develop premises to enable those people to be housed under one roof. General practice management changed to accommodate these different functions of managing a number of people, understanding how to organise the running of a building which was larger than a single house or surgery, in addition to looking after the doctor and undertaking the supportive functions.

In the 1980s, life moved on another step with the introduction of the New Contract, which brought with it health promotion and target payments for immunisations and vaccinations and cervical cytology. Once again, the practice management functions changed to incorporate the skills required to organise the workload and systems around maximising income through providing health promotion and ensuring targets were achieved. Next came the introduction of fundholding in 1991. For the first time, this gave general practitioners a direct ability to plan services for their entire population, for GMS, elective and community services, prescribing, and to purchase what was required. Fundholding reinforced needs assessment, introduced clinical guidelines between primary and secondary care, and allowed the primary healthcare team to consider how best to manage the patient through reinvesting resources into the area of care they felt was most necessary. In relation to these two areas came a whole new set of functions within the role of practice management, organising the writing and application for health promotion clinics, the organisation of cervical cytology recall and immunisation systems, business plans and auditable systems around the recording of activity and finance related to fundholding. In addition, health promotion and fundholding encouraged clinical guidelines which helped to support more diagnostic work in primary care and also encouraged good quality prescribing through practice formularies.

All these things needed to be managed, and with the increasingly complex range of functions was added the management of change, within the group of general practitioners, the primary healthcare team, and with secondary care clinicians and managers. Skills for a practice manager clearly changed and were much more related to:

- negotiation skills, ensuring a win/win situation both for consumer-related issues and contract outcomes;

- the management of change;

- financial and business planning;

- strategic planning: an ability to look into the future and plan over a number of years;

- an ability to 'hold the ring' for a large number of people and services (from my own background, I was at one time managing 68 individuals both from primary and secondary care who provided services to the practice population of 20 000);

- understanding of team building and team working;

▶ good communication skills at all levels, including direct with patients/clients, with colleagues within the primary healthcare team, with those within the Health Authority and Region, with provider organisations such as community and secondary care and, in some cases, with the local authority; and

▶ awareness of good employment practices, recruitment and retention, reimbursement, etc.

The 1990s manager was a very different person from Dr Cameron's Janet of yesteryear.

Box 8.1.	Practice management development.
Janet:	Organising and managing the doctor's life including cooking meals and cleaning the home
Mrs Findlay:	Answered calls and triaged, gave advice
1960s:	Health Centre management Managing people
1980s:	Developing systems for target payments Health Promotion Clinics
1990s:	Negotiation skills, ensuring a win/win situation The management of change Financial and business planning Strategic planning An ability to 'hold the ring' Understanding of team building and team working Good communication skills at all levels Awareness of good employment practices

Parallel to this, there has been a gradual movement within the general practitioner's role from the original Ballantyne model of the doctor and patient being the prime relationship, to the doctor and the practice population and, much more recently with the advent of the Primary Care Group (PCG), an emphasis on the doctor and the total local population. Practice managers have mirrored this change.

So why have practice managers? It would seem most of the reason for having practice managers was, and still is, to allow general practitioners to work as clinicians.

Future functions and structure of primary care

There are a number of changes which have occurred towards the end of the 1990s which have changed some of the functions within primary care management (note the subtle shift of description from 'practice' to 'primary care'). The twenty-first century is adding to the already large range of issues a host of new areas for primary care to tackle, including:

- clinical governance;

- multiple clinicians in the primary health care team, including general practitioners, nurse practitioners, practice nurses, district nurses, health visitors, counsellors, clinical psychologists, physiotherapists, speech therapists, etc.;

- a need to have the appropriate skill mix within the primary healthcare team;

- a flexibility to respond to outside demands, either made nationally through National Service Frameworks, throughout a health authority such as Health Improvement Programme issues, and primary care group issues within the Primary Care Investment Plan;

- professional development plans and practice development plans;

- financial and numerical skills to bid for money outside the NHS;

- partnership working; and

- information management and technology.

There seems to be a natural change which is occurring within some of the more well-developed practices to divide this work into pure administration of the service, i.e. appointments, response to patients, financial accountability, etc. and service development, e.g. supporting the development of personal development plans, practice development plans, application for individual sums of money through the Modernisation Fund, and input into areas of work such as 'Sure Start' (the government's programme to support the evolution of generic and holistic development for areas with very poor health and achievement through education; particularly levelled at 0–4 year olds and their parents) and urban regeneration.

At the same time, primary care groups are looking towards primary care trust status. It is likely that primary care trusts will bring together primary care as we know it, with our community colleagues, i.e. district nurses, health visitors, speech therapists, physios, etc. and wherever possible some local authority colleagues. It might be easier at this point to look at a number of models of primary care based on these functions, and which I hope will paint a more robust picture of what I have been describing (Figure 8.1).

Model of the 1990s

At this time there were two distinctions within general practice. In one model there was the singleton general practice with all general practitioners in it as independent contractors responsible for the provision of GMS services to their practice population. The Health Authority were responsible for commissioning all secondary and tertiary care, including mental health, and accountable for general medical services, quality and financial viability. Within the other model for the 1990s was still the singleton general practice with general practitioners having independent contractor status, but

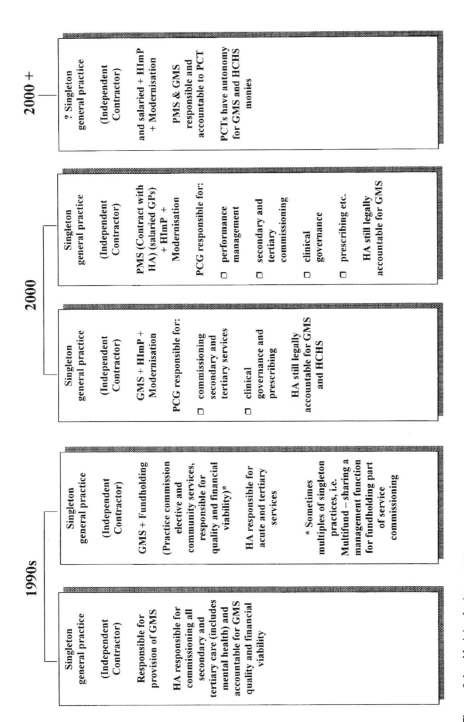

Figure 8.1. Models of primary care.

these people were responsible both for providing the GMS services and hospital and community services under the fundholding scheme. The practice commissioned elective hospital and community services and were responsible for quality and financial viability (sometimes these practices worked in multiples of singleton practices, i.e. through a multifund, sharing a management function for the fundholding part of service commissioning). The Health Authority remained responsible for acute and tertiary services other than those within the fundholding scheme.

Models for 2000

Again, there is the singleton general practice with independent contractors within it. These people are responsible for the provision of services through GMS plus the implementation of the Health Improvement Programme and Modernising the NHS. The PCG is responsible for commissioning secondary and tertiary services, implementing clinical governance, and prescribing. The Health Authority is still legally accountable for GMS and hospital and community health services. The other model for the current year is of singleton general practices and independent contractor doctors within them, but this time there is a personal medical services pilot (the practice contracts with the Health Authority for general medical services and includes the ability to have salaried general practitioners). They are also responsible for the implementation of the Health Improvement Programme and NHS Modernisation. The PCG remains responsible for performance management of the PMS contract, secondary and tertiary commissioning, clinical governance, and prescribing. The Health Authority still remains legally accountable for general medical services under the PMS scheme.

Model for 2001+

This is where there is some question as to the ability for practices to remain working singly, and whether the independent contractor status will remain. General practitioners could be salaried and will still be responsible for the implementation of the Health Improvement Programmes and the Modernisation of the NHS. PMS and GMS functions will remain, and the responsibility and accountability will be to the Primary Care Trust. Primary Care Trusts have autonomy for GMS and hospital and community health services monies. They may also employ all clinicians within the service provision of general medical services, as they are both commissioners and providers.

Requirements of practice management in The New NHS

It would seem likely that primary care trusts will cover the country within the next 2–5 years. In essence they will bring together the management of primary care and community services. They may in some cases go even further than this to include some social care provided through the local authorities at the present time, and possibly mental health.

Managers in primary care will need to be able to:

▶ provide the capacity to manage multiple clinicians, both primary care (general practice and community services) and, in some cases, secondary care;

▶ implement clinical governance, in particular ensuring that clinical guidelines are adhered to, through audit review and restructuring of services dependent on audit, taking corrective action where necessary, to ensure effective critical incident reporting;

▶ achieve good practice in terms of streamlining employment, terms and conditions, etc.;

▶ manage the development of care pathways around issues such as chronic disease management with secondary care colleagues and, where necessary, local authority and voluntary sector organisations;

▶ manage activity and finance;

▶ support the applications for things which come our way, through modernisation monies, lottery money, etc.;

▶ continue to be an agent of change;

▶ encompass the practical implementation of IM&T and the local Information for Health strategy (LIfH);

▶ continue to be an excellent communicator throughout all sectors, including our local population;

▶ be a negotiator where the outcome is win/win; and

▶ ensure access to services through a well-run general practice/primary care organisation.

For this to happen I foresee more separation of administrative and service development and two types of manager required to deliver the services. This will be further influenced by the need to streamline managers in general practice and community trusts as the primary care trusts emerge and remove the need for duplication of managers and raise questions of efficiency in relation to size of organisation and management capacity, i.e. do you need one development-style manager per 3000 patients?

In order for the PCT to happen, I believe general practice must have the following:

▶ Ownership of the system.

▶ Empowerment within the processes set up.

▶ Control of the situation, particularly in relation to their clinical care.

▶ Understanding that they have fair shares in things through open and transparent working (staffing levels, etc.).

Box 8.2. 2000 and beyond.

▶ Multiple clinicians

▶ Skill mix – effective and efficient resource utilisation

▶ Clinical governance

▶ Good practice for employment (PCT)

▶ Develop care pathways

▶ Boundary breakers

▶ Financial acumen

▶ Flexibility to respond/bids, etc.

▶ Professional and practice development plans

▶ Ppartnership working

▶ IM&T

▶ Change agent

▶ Communication ++

▶ Negotiation win/win

▶ Ensure access to services – well run, etc.

▶9

Self-management

Rifat Atun

Introduction

The National Health Service in Britain has recently been subject to a new set of reform initiatives. The White Paper *The New NHS. Modern. Dependable* (DoH 1998) can be seen as the logical conclusion to the reforms started in the 1980s. The wave of reforms began with the Griffiths Report (Griffiths 1983), followed by *Working for Patients* (DoH 1989) and the primary care-led NHS initiative (NHS Executive 1994).

The 1998 White Paper (DoH 1998) has established primary care as the platform for development not at the margins but at the heart of the health system and has brought the system nearer to the patient.

The outcome of the latest round of reforms is the reinforcement of the commissioner–provider focus, further decentralisation of commissioning, planning, and financial management functions and devolution of decision-making to primary care level. This has been accompanied by new frameworks for performance and accountability to ensure more homogeneous standards of quality and a greater responsiveness to the users' needs.

It can be argued that there is no significant deviation from the trajectory of polices of the last government. However, the new White Paper formalises the development of mechanisms to contain costs, maintain quality and improve accountability of not just the management but also the health professionals within the system.

Past policies have oscillated between establishing regulatory and market mechanisms and so improving the efficiency and effectiveness of the system. The pendulum seems to have swung convincingly towards regulation at the expense of market forces.

The new White Paper, as the name suggests, has 'modern' and 'modernisation' at its heart, although it is not clear exactly what is meant by these terms. It remains to be seen, however, how far these policies will be translated into practice. Within this 'modernisation' agenda a significant emphasis is placed on 'innovation'. The focal point of this thrust seems to be primary care, but where will the funding come from for this initiative?

So what are the implications of these policy changes for the young GP? Their impact cannot be ascertained in isolation without considering wider changes in the health care environment. A close examination of the health care environment is warranted as this will allow appreciation of the interplay of the forces that are shaping the health sector.

Analysis of the health care environment

The environmental analysis can be undertaken using the PEST model. It allows an analysis of the changes and trends in the political, economic, socio-demographic, and technological domains. Table 9.1 summarises some of the key drivers in the health care environment.

Table 9.1. Environmental analysis using PEST framework.

Domain of analysis	Drivers	Likely impact on the health sector and GPs
Political	Modernisation of the state	Efficiency drive
	Greater accountability (clinical governance, commission for health improvement)	Reduced autonomy
		Greater emphasis on performance management
		Need to justify a return on investments
	Public–private partnerships	Increased public scrutiny and involvement
	Value for money initiatives	in decision making
	Empowerment of users	Challenge to the authority of professionals
Economic	Rising incomes but also rising inequalities	Epidemiological polarisation
		Demand and supply mismatch
	Increased cost of health care provision	Priority setting and explicit rationing
	Budgetary squeeze	
Socio-demographic	Demographic transition	Ageing population
	Epidemiological transition	Chronic disease prevalent
	Changing value systems	Consumer society
	Changing public expectations	Increased focus on 'self' and less on community
		Increased litigation
Technological	New medical technology	Increased cost of health care delivery
	Internet revolution	Increased availability of timely information to users
		Profession's monopoly on information reduced

The new primary care

The interaction of the drivers for change and the accompanying policy thrust translates into a rather turbulent and dynamic health care environment. Within this rapidly changing environment the traditional approaches and possession of a limited set of core (and mainly clinical) skills are no longer adequate, nor appropriate. Many GPs whose skill base is limited to a core set of clinical know-how find that this is woefully inadequate to the challenges and demands of the new context. This inadequacy is in part due to the failure of many GPs in the last 10 years to respond adequately to a dynamic and rapidly changing environment and in part to the cushioning effect provided by an outdated National Contract. The impact of this has been a misunderstanding of what primary care really is.

Primary care has been considered by many (on both the regulatory and provider

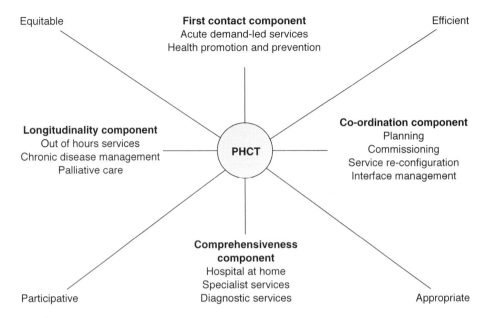

Figure 9.1. Primary healthcare.

sides of the fence) to be a set of activities, described in the Red Book, and delivered by a number of professionals bound by sets of rigid job descriptions and roles. The presence of this culture fuelled by a central contract has encouraged rigid working practices, entrenchment of professional groups, fragmentation of the care processes and a wasteful duplication of effort. A visible lack of incentives for development encouraged a minimalist attitude and fostered an environment that penalised innovation.

However, the scene has changed. Primary care is no longer viewed by the policy makers as a static set of activities but a dynamic domain within the health system. It is the domain for the first contact. It has moved beyond the traditional 'gatekeeper' role to being the co-ordinator of the health system. Improved training and teamwork has seen the development of more comprehensive services and care processes enhancing continuity (Figure 9.1).

New primary care, new competences

New primary care brings with it a new set of requirements, a new set of core competences for the organisation and the professionals within it.

In addition, the new dynamism and complexity, driven by changes in the environment and government policies, has established a system that is not suitable for management through regulation but to flexible organisational structures. These structures need to be managed by a new breed of professionals, who can manage

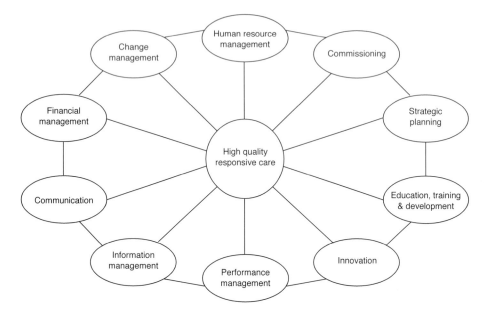

Figure 9.2. The competence framework.

complex organisational networks, and respond rapidly to changes. This requires a new set of skills and competences that foster diversity, innovation and continuous improvement both at individual and organisational level. This is in contrast to those entrenched in the outmoded traditional roles prevailing in the NHS.

For the young GP in this new environment a set of core competences is needed and represent an addition to the traditional set of clinical and 'doctoring' skills. These competences are outlined in Figure 9.2.

In management literature the term core competence has its origins in economics and strategic management. Prahalad and Hamel (1990) define core competences for an organisation as 'the collective learning in the organisations, especially how to co-ordinate diverse production skills and integrate multiple streams of technologies'. These competences are seen as the source to sustainable competitive advantage but to be so they need to exhibit a number of characteristics:

▶ They will be unique to the organisation.

▶ They will be sustainable because they are hard to imitate or substitute.

▶ They will offer some functionality to the customer.

▶ They will be partly the product of learning and will hence incorporate tacit as well as explicit knowledge (Nonaka and Takeuchi 1995).

▶ They will be generic, finding their way into a number of products and/or processes.

▶ They will take time to build.

Competition is much frowned upon in the NHS and although the new environment has reduced competition between organisations, it has created a competitive environment between professionals working in the primary care system, namely managers, GPs and the rest of the primary care team. Emergence of new structures (NHS Direct), and health professionals (nurse consultants, community pharmacists), is eroding the traditional role of the GP. Young GPs have to respond to this challenge by considering where they 'add value' in the system and where the non-value-added work can be delegated or transferred to other team members. This means identifying and occupying a new niche for themselves to ensure they survive into the future. As the young GP will be operating in a dynamic and not a static environment this position and niche needs to be reviewed and renewed regularly. This requires 'Self-management', a systematic and co-ordinated approach to managing and controlling one's growth and development.

The recipe for effective 'self-management' contains four ingredients, namely:

▶ Being entrepreneurial.

▶ Having a dynamic portfolio of skills and competences.

▶ Learning to manage.

▶ Using effective time management.

The entrepreneurial GP

To operate effectively and responsively within this dynamic health care environment the young GP and the organisations within which they work need to be entrepreneurial (Table 9.2).

There is much confusion about what is meant by being 'entrepreneurial'. Many associate this term with commerce or private sector business, just as many associated purchaser–provider split with privatisation. Contrary to popular belief being entrepreneurial does not necessarily involve working in the private sector. It is possible to be an entrepreneur within public sector institutions.

Table 9.2. The six dimensions of entrepreneurship (Stevenson 1997).

Dimension	Explanation
Strategic orientation	Being aware of the factors that drive an organisation's formulation of strategy
Commitment to opportunity	Identifying opportunities in the 'Environment' and not being constrained by resources in hand
Commitment of resources	Ability to maximise value creation by commitment of appropriate resources necessary to pursue a given opportunity
Control of resources	Ability to use own and other's resources; this refers to employing or outsourcing some resources
Management structures	Good co-ordination of key-controlled and non-controlled resources, developing favourable culture, flexibility and networking
Reward philosophy	More explicit focus on value creation and once created harvesting this value to benefit of all stakeholders

Generally, entrepreneurs are achievement oriented, like to take responsibility for decisions and dislike repetitive, routine work (Kets de Vries 1997). Creative entrepreneurs possess high levels of energy and perseverance. They are imaginative, with a willingness to take calculated risks to enable them to transform ideas into something concrete. They are not, as many conceive, gamblers. They are, however, a heterogeneous group and come from all walks of life.

To the organisation they convey a sense of purpose and determination and convince others where the action is. They tend to have leadership qualities and give their organisations a momentum. They tend to pull their organisation towards the entrepreneurial spectrum of management as opposed to stifling bureaucracy or administration. Other factors that push or pull an organisation away from a bureaucratic and an administrative setting towards the entrepreneurial end of the spectrum are those that force the organisation to:

▶ Be action oriented.

▶ Have short decision windows.

▶ Manage risk.

▶ Have limited decision constituencies.

This is in contrast to factors that enforce an administrative behaviour. These include:

▶ Multiple decision constituencies.

▶ Pressure for consensus making and having to negotiate strategy.

▶ An environment that aims to reduce risk.

▶ Managing resources and 'projects' to ensure participation of existing players.

Clearly, the factors in the former scenario are reminiscent of those prevailing in general practice as a small organisation. Those factors in the latter scenario are more suggestive of an environment prevailing in health authorities or perhaps their new offspring, the Primary Care Group (PCG) or Primary Care Trust (PCT).

The health care environment is dynamic and turbulent. To innovate and be responsive the young GP has to balance the administrative pull generated by the new structures in the NHS, such as the PCGs or PCTs.

Managing a portfolio of competences

To flourish in a changing and dynamic environment it is necessary for the young GP to renew his/her competences, managing a portfolio of resources and competences. However, one should differentiate between different kinds of competences ranging from threshold to unique competences. Examples of each are outlined in Table 10.3.

Threshold competences are those that will be possessed by all GP principals. These are the 'minimum qualifying criteria' that enable a GP to practise as a principal and become a 'practitioner' following acquisition of basic medical knowledge and skills at medical school and vocational training schemes.

Table 9.3. Link to competitive advantage.

Attribute	GP example
Threshold competences	Clinical skills
	Basic medical knowledge
Unique competences	Ability to manage effectively
	Efficiency
	New services

On the other hand, unique competences will differentiate the possessor and confer a distinct competitive advantage to self and to the organisation. These competences range from generic management skills that enable the GP to develop new services to specialist clinical skills that enable the development of a value-added clinical service.

Many GPs will never move beyond the threshold competence level. Those who develop unique competences are the entrepreneurial GPs who will scan the horizon for new developments, anticipate trends and position themselves and their organisations to reap the benefits (Figure 9.3).

Horizon scanning is important as this may yield valuable intelligence on future trends and enable the GP to prepare appropriate skills and competences in areas where there is likely to be market growth and development. This scanning and analysis of trends will guide GPs to renew and refresh the portfolio of competences necessary to respond to opportunities.

The focus should be on areas where there is likely to be growth and opportunity for development and where this is a strategic fit with the individual and organisational values, priorities, and competences.

In the dynamic health care sector there are many sub-sectors and market segments where there is likely to be scope for significant growth (Atun 1998). The opportunities should not be underestimated and so a young GP can broaden his/her vision and be entrepreneurial.

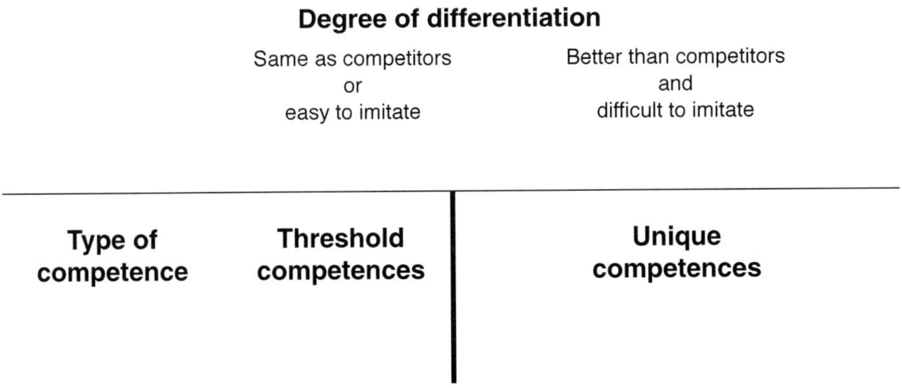

Degree of differentiation

	Same as competitors or easy to imitate	Better than competitors and difficult to imitate
Type of competence	**Threshold competences**	**Unique competences**

Figure 9.3. Managing the portfolio.

GP and management

General management was introduced in the NHS in 1983 following the recommendations of the Griffiths Report. Since then the number and strength of managers has increased inexorably. In the highly managerial world of the health sector there are two options for the young GP: learn to manage or be managed. The former option is clearly preferable as the latter option would leave GPs vulnerable to managerial pressures. Furthermore, young GPs have much to add to management in the Health Service (Atun 1997).

However, many GPs are not comfortable with the idea of being involved in management. This may be in part due to their perception that management conflicts with 'professional' duties. Mintzberg (1990), in an elegant article, described the 'job of the manager' which yielded remarkable similarities to that of a GP. Indeed, both jobs consist of similar activities albeit with differing names (Atun 1999). Given these demonstrable similarities it can be argued that a GP's role naturally prepares him/her to take on management duties. What is necessary is to make not just a professional but a mental transition in the way we think of management and see how we apply management principles in everyday practice.

GP involvement in management is necessary to change the way health care organisations function. In particular the young GP should learn and aim to:

▶ Reduce bureaucracy/politics.

▶ Manage organisation-wide for cohesion.

▶ Manage across organisations with partners.

▶ Get things done speedily.

▶ Delegate.

Time management

Effective self-management requires effective time management. Time is a valuable and a scarce resource which people spend ineffectively. One can have some control over how this resource is spent and ensure it is not wasted. This will involve making choices. Recognising this is the first step on the path to effective time management.

Much time is wasted because of failure to recognise and eliminate common 'time robbers' due to having unclear priorities and spending too much time on unimportant matters, repeated interruptions, an unwillingness to say 'no', wasting excessive time in meetings, and procrastination.

Poor time management is a source of stress and a barrier to effective self-management. The way to improve time management is by observing the 12 golden rules, namely:

1. Make a 'to do' list with ranking of priorities and regular revision.
2. Identify priorities and distinguish between tasks that are urgent and tasks which are important (urgent tasks have an immediate impact. Important tasks have a significant impact).

3. Address top priorities when fresh and functioning at 'best' level. That means leaving routine and unimportant matters to times when tired.
4. Critically evaluate how to best use time.
5. Use small gaps productively.
6. Tackle big tasks in a piecemeal fashion and break them into small achievable tasks with clear deadlines.
7. Do more than one trivial task at a time.
8. Stop procrastination.
9. Do not defer decisions or actions. Aim to handle a paper or a message once and do not hoard.
10. Use time released pro-actively.
11. Avoid vertical filing and creating paper heaps. Remember the motto 'A place for everything and everything in its place'.
12. To be an effective time manager adopt a rule per month and at the end of the year reflect on your achievements.

Conclusions

Effective self-management involves being entrepreneurial, developing and renewing a portfolio of competences, being an effective manager and organising your time.

The recipe for success lies in developing not just a knowledge base in clinical specialties, but an array of social, entrepreneurial and managerial skills with appropriate attitudes to face the challenges before us. These are the building blocks collectively needed for effective self-management. Knowledge of the functional areas and having a limited and a static set of skills is no longer enough. The young GP needs an armamentarium of competences that are renewed and refreshed.

The art of self-management is the development and application of these competences just as good clinical practice is the art of applying medical science. This means being able to learn from the past, innovate in the present, and anticipate for the future.

References

Atun R A (1997). Should doctors manage or be manage? *Clinician in Management*, **6**: 6–13.
Atun R A (1998). Opportunities in the UK health care market. A strategic analysis. Financial Times Health Care Reports. *Financial Times*. May.
Atun R A (1999). Demystifying management. *Clinician in Management* **8**: 47–50.
Department of Health (1989). *Working for Patients*. London: HMSO.
Department of Health (1998). *New NHS. Modern. Dependable*. London: HMSO.
Griffiths R (1983). *NHS Management Inquiry: Report*. London: DHSS.
Kets de Vries M (1997). Creative rebels with a cause. In: Birley S, Muzyka D F (eds). *Mastering Enterprise*. London: Financial Times.
Mintzberg H (1990). The manager's job: folklore and fact. *Harvard Business Review*. **March–April**: 163–176.
NHS Executive (1994). *Primary Care-Led NHS*. EL (94) 79.
Nonaka I, Takeuchi H (1995). *The Knowledge-creating Company: How Japanese Companies Create the Dynamics of Innovation*. New York: Oxford University Press.
Prahalad C K, Hamel G (1990). The core competence of the corporation. *Harvard Business Review* **68**: 79–91.
Stevenson H (1997). Six dimensions of entrepreneurship. In: Birley S, Muzyka D F (eds) *Mastering Enterprise*. London: Financial Times.

▶10

Medical, Legal and Ethical Challenges

Gerard Panting

Confidence in doctors is at an all time low. The fallout from the Ledward and Shipman cases has tainted the entire profession, placing accountability firmly at the top of the agenda at the General Medical Council, Department of Health and for every newspaper, pundit and politician. Medical practice and the environment in which doctors must work is more challenging than ever. So what can doctors do to avoid the numerous pitfalls of practice?

There is no foolproof answer but the chances of being subjected to substantial criticism can be minimised by being aware of your legal and professional responsibilities, exercising sound clinical judgement, ensuring good communication with both patients and other health care professionals, administering your practice competently and maintaining adequate medical records.

Legal responsibilities

Medical practice is regulated by a mixture of statute (Acts of Parliament and Statutory Instruments), common law based upon judgments handed down by the courts at the conclusion of specific cases and the guidance promulgated by the General Medical Council. The legal aspects of medical practice described in this chapter reflect English law. The law in Scotland, Northern Ireland, the Isle of Man and the Channel Islands is broadly similar but differs in some respects.

In particular, doctors need to know about: consent and confidentiality, complaints and disciplinary procedures, the GMC, the role of the Coroner and writing medico-legal reports. However, there are many other legal aspects of medical practice and, if you are unsure about how best to proceed in a particular instance, always check with someone who knows before rather than after the event.

Consent

Consent is a fundamental principle of medical law, protecting the competent individual's right to autonomy. To embark on any examination, investigation or treatment without valid consent amounts to battery and/or negligence and may result in civil or criminal proceedings, or both.

For consent to treatment to be valid, the patient must be competent, have sufficient information to make an informed choice and consent freely to the procedure or treatment.

It is generally assumed that adult patients are competent, but this is not always the case. The test is whether the individual can understand the implications of accepting or rejecting the proposed treatment and available alternatives. If so, the patient is competent and (unless the Mental Health Act applies) his or her wishes must be respected even if, from an objective point of view, they are irrational or likely to cause serious harm or even death.

But patients cannot be expected to make a decision unless they have sufficient information to make a choice. The question is how much information is sufficient? Last year, the GMC published *Seeking Patients' Consent: The Ethical Considerations.* Box 10.1, taken from that booklet, sets out the information which patients want or

---

Box 10.1. What patients need to know before giving consent.

▶ Details of the diagnosis and prognosis, and the likely prognosis if the condition is left untreated.

▶ Uncertainties about the diagnosis including options for further investigation prior to treatment.

▶ Options for treatment or management of the condition, including the option not to treat.

▶ The purpose of a proposed investigation or treatment; details of the procedures or therapies involved, including subsidiary treatment such as methods of pain relief; how the patient should prepare for the procedure; and details of what the patient might experience during or after the procedure including common and serious side-effects.

▶ For each option, explanations of the likely benefits and the probabilities of success; and discussion of any serious or frequently occurring risks, and of any lifestyle changes which may be caused by, or necessitated by, the treatment.

▶ Whether a proposed treatment is experimental.

▶ How and when the patient's condition and any side-effects will be monitored or re-assessed.

▶ The name of the doctor who will have overall responsibility for the treatment and, where appropriate, names of the senior members of his or her team.

▶ Whether doctors in training will be involved, and the extent to which students may be involved in an investigation or treatment.

▶ A reminder that patients can change their minds about a decision at any time.

▶ A reminder that patients have a right to seek a second opinion.

▶ Where applicable, details of costs or changes which the patient may have to meet.

---

ought to know before deciding whether to consent to treatment or an investigation. GMC guidance applies throughout the UK.

Consent can only be valid if it is given freely. Coercing a patient into a decision, failing to give the patient time to mull over the options or misrepresenting the situation may all lead to sustainable allegations that the consent was invalid.

Children, that is patients under 16 years of age, who can understand the implications of proposed treatment, can also be competent to give consent. Although in many circumstances involvement of the parent or guardian is advisable, any situation where a child seeks medical care while refusing to tell a parent can pose considerable difficulty and it is always best to seek advice if you are unsure as how best to proceed.

But not all patients are competent. Anyone with parental responsibility may consent on behalf of an incompetent minor (anyone under 18 years of age) and in an emergency, with no-one available to consent on behalf of a minor, the doctor should do whatever is necessary to protect the best interests of his patient in the absence of consent.

No-one, not even the courts, can consent on behalf of an incompetent adult so in these cases the doctor must act in the best interests of the patient as determined by a responsible body of medical opinion. The only exception to the 'best interests' rule is where the patient is competent and has made an advance directive or living will specific to the current circumstances, expressly prohibiting certain forms of treatment.

The same principles apply in situations of fluctuating capacity. When incompetent, the patient should be treated according to his or her best interests unless this conflicts with an advance directive clearly stated by the patient when competent and applicable in the circumstances.

Consent to treatment may be express or implied. Where the nature and purpose of the procedure is self-evident and there is no risk of significant adverse effects, implied consent is all that is required. If, however, there is any significant risk, express consent should be obtained. This may be obtained orally or in writing. In general, consent forms are reserved for cases under general anaesthetic or more complex procedures. A signed consent form is, at best, only some evidence that valid consent has been obtained. In the event of any complaint or claim, it is likely to be the amount of information given to the patient which is the determining factor in deciding whether or not that consent was valid.

Patients can be compulsorily detained for assessment and/or treatment under various sections of the Mental Health Act (1983) (England and Wales) even in the face of express refusal. Broadly equivalent statutes apply elsewhere. The sections most relevant to GPs are set out in Box 10.2.

Compulsory treatment under the Mental Health Act may include management of physical consequences of a mental disorder. For example, a patient suffering from anorexia nervosa and consequently vulnerable to physical harm through malnutrition may be treated with appropriate nutrition against his or her will. Similarly, a patient suffering from depression who has taken an overdose of paracetamol may be treated for the physical consequences of the paracetamol overdose if the conditions for compulsory detention are met.

Box 10.2. Mental Health Act 1983 (England and Wales).

Section 2	This section authorises the compulsory detention of a patient for up to 28 days. Two medical recommendations are required, one from a practitioner approved under Section 12 of the Act, usually a consultant psychiatrist, and a second from a doctor with a previous acquaintance of the patient, usually the patient's own family doctor.
	Patients may be detained under Section 2 if they pose a threat to their own health or safety or to the health and safety of others and they are suffering from a mental disorder of a nature or degree which warrants detention of the patient in hospital for assessment.
	Drug or alcohol dependence are not, in themselves, considered to be mental disorders justifying compulsory admission.
Section 3	*Admission for treatment*
	The procedure is similar to that under Section 2 but the practitioners making the recommendation must be of the opinion that medical treatment in hospital is appropriate.
Section 4	This may only be used in genuine emergencies where it is not possible to obtain a second medical recommendation to support an application under Section 2. The medical recommendation is made by one doctor, preferably with previous knowledge of the patient, usually the general practitioner.
	The patient must then be admitted to hospital within 24 hours and may be detained for up to 72 hours unless detention under Section 2 or 3 is effected.

Complaints

Complaints are a fact of professional life. Every doctor can expect to receive some complaints during the course of a career.

The vast majority of complaints are resolved at local resolution level. This is the informal, often practice-based or Health Authority facilitated conciliation part of the complaints procedure which aims to bring complaints to a quick conclusion.

Where something has gone wrong, patients are entitled to a clear explanation of exactly what has happened and there is certainly no need to shy away from apologising if the investigation reveals some shortcoming on the part of the practice. The golden rules of complaints handling are set out in Box 10.3.

If local resolution fails, the complainant is entitled to apply for an independent review of the complaint. Applications are vetted by a lay, non-executive director of the Health Authority (in England and Wales), termed the Convenor, who must decide whether all that can be done has been achieved at local resolution level and whether an independent review would add anything further to the process.

> **Box 10.3.** Golden rules of complaint handling.
>
> 1. Ensure that you understand exactly what the complainant is dissatisfied about.
>
> 2. Explain the system so that the complainant knows who is dealing with their complaint and when a response can be expected.
>
> 3. Investigate the facts before attempting to explain what has happened.
>
> 4. If the complainant is not the patient, ensure that appropriate authority has been obtained before divulging any confidential information.
>
> 5. Do not be afraid to apologise where something has gone wrong.
>
> 6. Do not be afraid to make concessions where the patient makes a good point during the complaint process.
>
> 7. Do not accept incorrect or inaccurate statements simply to bring the procedure to an end: it probably will not and withdrawing concessions undermines any trust the complainant may have in you.
>
> 8. Include in your response any lessons the practice feels it has learnt from the complaint and how recognised deficiencies are to be rectified.
>
> 9. Remember that the complaints procedure is consumer-orientated. If it does not address the complainant's need it is doomed to failure.
>
> 10. If the patient remains dissatisfied, tell them how to pursue their complaint to the Health Authority.

Comparatively few, just 1–2% of complaints, are accepted for independent review which is a more formal process working to specific terms of reference. The lay chairman has considerable discretion on how the Panel operates. In some, both complainant and respondent will be present throughout. In others, members will interview all involved sequentially. At the conclusion of the investigation, the Panel produces a report made available to the parties and the Health Authority, which may include recommendations.

Complainants dissatisfied with a Convenor's refusal to admit a complaint for independent review or with the outcome of an independent review may ask the Health Service Commissioner (or Ombudsman) to review the handling of their complaint. The Ombudsman can, if he sees fit, take over the entire investigation of the complaint or require the Health Authority to reconsider the case.

The Coroner

The post of Coroner dates back to Norman times. The original role was to ensure that all monies due to the Crown following various forms of unnatural death were collected and not misappropriated locally. The only fiscal aspect of the role which remains is the determination of Treasure Trove. The modern day Coroner's responsibility is to identify who has died, where and when they died and by what means. By convention, doctors decline to write a death certificate in any case where there is no obvious cause of death or where the death is not due to natural causes.

Box 10.4 sets out the circumstances in which death should be reported to the Coroner.

Box 10.4. The Registrar (of deaths) must report a death when:

▶ No doctor attended the deceased during the last illness.

▶ There is no medical certificate of cause of death.

▶ The deceased was not attended by a doctor in the last 14 days of life.

▶ The cause of death is unknown or is believed to have been unnatural, caused by violence or neglect, or abortion.

▶ Death occurred in suspicious circumstances.

▶ Death occurred during an operation or on recovery from the anaesthetic.

▶ When death resulted from industrial disease or poisoning.

Curiously, at present, there is no statutory obligation on a doctor to report a death to the Coroner. A change in the law, however, seems likely post-Harold Shipman.

In addition, Coroners may have their own local requirements which hospitals and GPs should be aware of and satisfy.

At a Coroner's inquest, interested parties may be legally represented. In many cases, legal representation is not required but, should the family of the deceased be legally represented or the Coroner raises concerns over the patient's care or the doctor feels vulnerable to criticism, or the press shows considerable interest, serious consideration should be given to legal representation of the doctor.

Writing medico-legal reports

Writing medico-legal reports is another inescapable facet of modern medical practice. Before putting pen to paper, the doctor should ensure that there is appropriate authority, e.g. the patient's consent, to disclose that information.

The exact form of the report will depend upon the circumstances but it is usual to start with some information about yourself and your practice (when you qualified, how long you have been in your current post, previous experience relevant to the subject matter of the report, etc.). Next, set out the facts relevant to the report. If it concerns your management of a patient's care, you should write the report in the first person singular so that there is no confusion about who did what and when. Ensure that your own action is placed in context by recording the history in strict chronological order and including relevant actions of others, albeit a more detailed account of their involvement will be set out in their own report. On completion of the report, read through it and, if there is any prospect of criticism of your own conduct, seek advice before submitting it.

Whatever the circumstances, the report must be accurate. Signing off a report known to be inaccurate, misleading or incorrect can result in severe criticism by the GMC (see below) and may result in loss of registration.

General Medical Council

The General Medical Council was established in 1858 primarily to enable the public to distinguish between registered (and therefore properly qualified) medical practitioners and the numerous quacks of the time.

From the outset, the GMC has had disciplinary powers, the ultimate sanction being erasure from the Medical Register. Doctors behaving badly always attract the media and so it is not surprising that the GMC is best known for its conduct procedures but this is just a small fraction of its work.

The GMC's core functions are:

▶ Maintaining an up-to-date register of qualified doctors.

▶ Fostering good medical practice.

▶ Promoting high standards of medical education.

▶ Protecting the public from doctors whose fitness to practise is in doubt.

The number of complaints made to the GMC is rising. In 1998, there were just 3000 complaints (against a total working population of 100 000 doctors in the UK). On average formal action will be taken in 600 cases with only 50 or so doctors appearing before the Conduct Committee every year.

The Register

The most important change in registration has been the introduction of the Specialist Register which enables the public and employers to know which doctors have completed an approved programme of higher specialist training. The Specialist Training Authority operating under the auspices of the Royal Colleges awards certificates for completion of specialist training, making the doctor eligible for inclusion in the Specialist Register which is now a prerequisite for an appointment to a substantive NHS consultant post.

Fostering good medical practice

The GMC produces a number of booklets that effectively set out standards which the Council expects individual doctors to follow. Of particular importance to doctors in training are:

- Good medical practice.
- Confidentiality.
- Serious communicable diseases.
- Consent: the ethical and legal issues.
- Recommendations on the training of specialists.

Promoting high standards of medical education

This applies to both undergraduate and postgraduate education. With regular visits to medical schools and through revalidation the GMC will, in due course, take an active interest in the continuing medical education and professional development of all registered medical practitioners.

Protecting the public from doctors whose fitness to practise is in doubt

The GMC operates three fitness to practise procedures:

- Conduct procedures.
- Health procedures.
- Performance procedures.

All complaints received by the GMC warranting further investigation are reviewed by members of Council termed Screeners. They decide if further action is required and, if so, which path that complaint should follow. Doctors are usually informed about complaints at an early stage and are offered the chance to comment before the papers are reviewed by the Screener. Should you receive a letter from the GMC ensure you take advice before attempting to respond.

Only a minority of cases are pursued beyond the screening stage.

Conduct procedures

Cases allocated to the conduct route are next considered by the Preliminary Proceedings Committee which currently meets in private and usually considers cases on the papers alone. Until July 2000 the PPC could, in certain circumstances, suspend or place conditions on a doctor's registration on an interim basis. This function has now been taken over by the new Interim Orders Committee.

The Preliminary Proceedings Committee decides which cases should be referred on to the PCC. The PCC meets in public and conducts the hearing very much like a trial with both prosecution and defence represented by lawyers, evidence given on oath and, if necessary, witnesses compelled to attend by subpoena.

Most cases are concluded within a day or two but some, like the Bristol and 'kidneys for sale' cases, last for weeks.

At the end of the hearing, the PCC considers first if the facts proved amount to serious professional misconduct and, if so, what sanctions should be applied. The options are:

▶ Admonishment.

▶ Conditions on the doctor's registration for up to three years.

▶ To suspend the doctor's name from the Medical Register for up to 12 month.

▶ To erase the doctor's name from the Medical Register (now for a minimum of five years).

Unlike the Conduct procedures, the Health and Performance procedures are designed to be remedial although the prime objective is always to protect patients.

The health procedures

Cases referred on for further investigation by the Health Screeners are dealt with relatively informally. The doctor is asked to undergo examination, usually by two doctors who then report their findings back to the Council. If necessary, the doctor will be asked to agree to the appointment of a medical supervisor who will report progress to the Council on a regular basis. Provided that the doctor agrees to co-operate and follows the various recommendations made (including medical treatment and restriction on medical practice) the case is unlikely to be referred to the Health Committee.

Doctors who do not comply or default from supervision are referred to the Health Committee which meets in private with the doctor present, together with appropriate legal representation.

The Health Committee can impose conditions on the doctor's registration for up to three years and suspend a doctor from the Medical Register for up to 12 months.

Performance procedures

The performance procedures are designed to deal with doctors who display a pattern of seriously deficient performance.

Where there is a suspicion that this is the case, doctors are invited to undergo an assessment by three assessors appointed by the Council – usually two doctors and one lay person. The assessment is comprehensive and lasts 2 or 3 days. It includes interviews with the doctor, observing the doctor in practice, interviews with professional colleagues, examination of patient records and examination-style questions. Following assessment, the assessors will submit a report to the Council which will report to a case co-ordinator with recommendations for correction of identified deficiencies. If these are serious, the doctor will be invited to agree to a statement of requirements intended to correct specific problems. Once that action has been taken, the doctor will be reassessed in the same way.

If doctors do not agree to an assessment, the case is considered by the Assessment Review Committee whose function is to determine whether or not there are grounds for an assessment.

The CPP considers only those cases where the doctor has refused to co-operate or where appropriate improvement has not been made within the programme.

The CPP may place conditions on the doctor's registration for up to 3 years, or suspend the doctor's registration for 12 months. Although the CPP cannot strike a doctor's name off the Register, they can suspend the doctor's name indefinitely once they have already suspended it for at least 2 years.

Confidentiality

The basic rule of confidentiality is straightforward. Patients have a right to expect that information about them will be held in confidence by their doctors. However, this apparently simple principle does generate complex problems which may be difficult to resolve, primarily because the duty is not absolute.

The GMC guidance on confidentiality sets out a number of exceptions where doctors may be able to justify or might be expected to breach professional confidence.

However, as stated in the final paragraph of their guidance, if you decide to disclose confidential information, you must be prepared to explain and justify your decision.

Holders of information about identifiable patients have a legal duty to ensure that it is protected against improper disclosure at all times.

The Data Protection Act 1998 sets out data protection principles (Box 10.5) which apply to data covered by the Act likely to include all health information held by general practitioners about their patients within practice filing systems, whether electronic or manual.

The exceptions to the general rule of confidentiality are: sharing information with the consent of the patient; sharing information with others providing care; disclosures that benefit patients indirectly; disclosure of identifiable information without consent; disclosure where doctors have dual responsibilities; disclosures without the patient's consent; disclosure in the interests of others; disclosure in the patient's medical interests where consent is unobtainable; disclosure after a patient's death.

Box 10.5.   Data protection principles.

Data must:

▶ Be obtained and processed fairly and lawfully.

▶ Be held for the lawful purposes described in the Data Users Register entry.

▶ Be adequate, relevant and not excessive in relation to the purposes for which they are held.

▶ Be accurate and, where necessary, kept up to date.

▶ Be held no longer than is necessary for the registered purposes.

▶ Be processed in accordance with the rights of the individual concerned to have information about themselves corrected or erased.

▶ Be surrounded by proper security and disclosed only to those people described in the Register entry.

▶ Not be transferred to countries outside the European economic area unless that country can ensure adequate protection for the rights and freedoms of the data subject.

Sound clinical practice

In the event of a complaint or claim, your defence is reliant upon demonstrating that you acted in accordance with acceptable medical practice. That process starts with putting yourself in a position to make a sound clinical judgement by taking a history, conducting an appropriate examination, initiating relevant investigations, etc. Managing the patient within established protocols or guidelines is obviously helpful when defending allegations of inadequate care. But guidelines may not exist or be applicable in every case; then you should be guided by established principles, where necessary, by reference to experienced colleagues and the relevant literature. (Legal assessment of cases is necessarily evidence-based so evidence-based practice has an in-built advantage.)

The communication net

A multitude of people may be involved in the care of any given patient, including the hospital team, the GP and his staff, the community nursing staff including perhaps special palliative care nurses, the social services department, the voluntary sector and the patient's family. Each member of the extended team must be aware of what they should be doing – which depends on all the left hands knowing what all the right hands are up to. That said, care must be taken not to breach confidentiality without proper justification.

Competent administration

Administration may be dull but efficient administration is, nevertheless, essential to any smooth running operation. Failure to provide appointments with appropriate expedition or at all is unacceptable, as is having no system in place to assess urgency or to check results, identify abnormalities and take necessary action, or simply failing to pass a simple message from a GP about a patient recently arrived in Casualty – 'By the way he's a diabetic.' A simple slip may have catastrophic results. Some administrative processes are extremely well worked out, e.g. marking the correct side for operation and swab counts in theatre, but in many hospitals systems are the result of evolution rather than design and may be over-dependent on assiduous attention to detail by one long-serving and loyal member of staff. What happens when that person goes sick or retires? Doctors are senior members of the team and must interest themselves in the mechanics of mundane processes.

Contemporaneous records

Complaints, claims of negligence and other forms of investigation may not materialise for weeks, months or even years after the events in question, by which time the doctor is unlikely to remember exactly what happened at a given consultation, particularly where there has been a sequence of consultations over a period of time. Even if only for corroboration, the doctor must be able to refer to contemporaneous medical records; if they are inadequate the doctor's position will be prejudiced.

One definition of an adequate medical record is one which enables the doctor to reconstruct the consultation without reference to memory, including: adequate details of the history; answers to relevant direct questions; a record of all systems examined, noting all positive findings and important negative findings as well as objective measurements such as blood pressure, peak flow, etc.; the clinical impression formed; any investigations ordered; treatment prescribed or referral made and arrangements for follow-up or admission.

Medical records should also be objective and worthy of independent scrutiny as, in the event of an investigation, the notes will be pored over in considerable detail.

Conclusion

The law governing medical practice cannot be summarised in 4500 words or even 45 000 words. If you need help, it is available from your medical defence society 24 hours a day so, if in doubt, do not hesitate to ask.

▶11

Transcultural Medicine

Bashir Qureshi

Introduction

Transcultural medicine means dealing with patients from different cultures. As people from every culture are strongly influenced by religious and ethnic biological make up, it is defined as follows:

'Transcultural Medicine is the knowledge of medical and communication encounters between a doctor or health worker of one ethnic group and a patient of another. It embraces the physical, psychological and social aspects of care as well as the scientific aspects of culture, religion and ethnicity without getting involved in the politics of segregation and integration' (Qureshi 1994).

The politics

Transcultural medicine is a new and politically sensitive subject because it pleads to health professionals for change in their caring attitudes while delivering medicine to their patients, from a mono-ethnic model of service to a multi-ethnic approach. Traditionally, the politics and economics of a nation have as much to do with medicine as disease. The one who pays the piper, calls the tune, and politicians are held responsible for the running of the National Health Service.

Politically, there has been a constant struggle between the forces of integration and segregation in every country and Britain is no exception. The integrationists encouraged the concept of Britain as a nation of individuals rather than groups; therefore, everyone is British. On the other hand, the segregationists demonstrate that the UK is a nation of diverse communities; therefore, everyone is English, Scottish, Welsh, Asian, Black or Chinese first. In 1948, when the NHS was founded, politicians urged doctors to practise medicine without regard to a patient's culture, religion or ethnicity. In 1992, recognising the change in British society by evolution, the patient's charter required NHS professionals to respect all patients' religious and cultural beliefs. The British courts have also taken note of this change. As I have been teaching the subject since 1981, I am particularly delighted that ethnic and transcultural issues have officially become one of the 17 core contents of the MRCGP examination since May 1998.

Box 11.1. The British nation today.

Cultures

Western, Eastern, Westernised Eastern

Religions

Hinduism, Buddhism, Sikhism, Judaism, Christianity, Islam
Persuasions (Liberalism, Secularism, Agnosticism, Atheism)

Ethnicities

Caucasians (Europeans, Middle Easterners), Asiatic (Asians), Negroid (Africans, Caribbeans), Mongoloid (Chinese)

Transcultural approach

While respecting integrationists and segregationists, let us move aside taking an objective look at today's British nation (Box 11.1). In keeping with other countries in the world, Britain has people from three cultures, six major world religions, four scientific persuasions, and four racial categories. Although the patients come from all the above 17 backgrounds, health care in Britain is mainly delivered by professionals who are either western or westernised easterners and hold liberal, secular or even agnostic persuasions. As the National Health Service is being gradually devolved to local primary care groups/trusts, politicians will increasingly monitor the appropriateness of health care for British citizens from the eastern culture, six religions and all four ethnic backgrounds. In fact, transcultural monitoring and transcultural medical litigations have already begun.

This chapter highlights the basic transcultural information a doctor or health professional needs to consider in making a diagnosis, in management and to achieve patient compliance (Box 11.2). It should help not only doctor–patient rapport in a transcultural contact but also reduce the chance of a failed consultation leading to a complaint or litigation.

Box 11.2. Patient's problems.

Physical	Cultural
Psychological	Religious
Social	Ethnic

A disease is caused by genetic and environmental factors, which are affected by:

▶ age, gender, social class, culture, religion, ethnicity.

Cultural influences

Culture means the customs and civilisation of a particular people or group. When a doctor comes from one culture and the patient from another, the following points should be considered without any hint of denigration to the patient.

Consultation attitudes

Western and westernised eastern patients would observe strict timing (within five minutes of a given time), an appointment system and a queue, no matter how long it may be. They would believe in the individual right of privacy, choice and responsibility. They would be used to sitting on committees with an agenda and reaching a consensus.

Eastern, non-westernised, patients would observe approximate timing (within an hour of given time), a demand-led consultation, allowing the needy to jump the queue. They would believe in shared privacy, shared choice and family responsibility. They would rather go to say prayers, have an open chat with the doctor or nurse and follow what they advise.

Make no mistake, whereas a western patient comes for consultation before making an informed decision, an eastern patient would come for advice and would accept a doctor or nurse's decision.

Verbal communication

It is vital for accurate history taking that the doctor and patient understand each other's language or the diagnosis may be wrongly made with serious consequences. An interpreter must be obtained, preferably from the Health Authority resources.

▶ Pain is the commonest symptom in medicine, particularly in general practice. The type of pain can be indicative of a particular disease (Box 11.3). However, a patient with a language barrier, and sometimes an interpreter, may not understand the difference between burning, gripping or stabbing pain because they may translate literally. In addition, three other cultural factors should be remembered:

> If a doctor were to ask 'Do you have gripping pain?', an eastern patient will not ask out of politeness:
> What do you mean doctor?
> I don't understand you, doctor!
> These are considered rude responses in the east.
>
> An easterner would not say 'I don't know' as it is frowned upon in the eastern culture.
>
> Out of frustration, so as to get out of the situation, he/she may say 'yes' which may be a wrong answer.

▶ Some words, e.g. cheat, have more serious meaning in the west than in the east.

Box 11.3. Verbal communication.

Pain – character

▶ Aching   (earache).

▶ Burning   (hiatus hernia).

▶ Gripping   (myocardial).

▶ Stabbing   (trigeminal nerve).

▶ Throbbing   (migraine).

▶ Colicky   (gut, renal).

▶ Gnawing   (peptic ulcer).

Non-verbal communication

Interpretation of good behaviour and gestures are different in various cultures and subcultures. Six areas of non-verbal communication must be understood so as to avoid repugnance in a medical consultation.

▶ Some east-European, Arab, and Asian, particularly Sri Lankan, names may be long, unpronounceable or have a rude sound in English (e.g. Fakir). Divide a long name into three or four syllables and ask the patient how to pronounce it. Never shorten names, without negotiating, as this may be considered an insulting or uncaring attitude.

▶ Some patients may get confused when facing a health professional from another racial background, especially for the first time. Recognise colour shock and negotiate.

▶ Sex segregation is advised by five major world religions: Judaism, Islam, Hinduism, Buddhism and Sikhism. Both men and women would need an acceptable arrangement.

▶ If an eastern patient is nodding his or her head more than four times in agreement, then probably the doctor and patient communication has broken down. Moreover, some Hindus nod their heads transversely as a sign of respect but it could be misunderstood as saying 'no'.

▶ Sign language can be a cause of instant repugnance. Readers would probably be aware of the meanings in the western culture; they should note that in the eastern culture, *it is very rude*:

  – to have constant eye contact. It means anger or an invitation for a date for a night out.
  – to show a finger and thumb circle. It means a threat of sexual abuse in public.
  – to show a thumbs up sign, it means 'up your . . .'.

Specific customs

▶ French patients may expect a medication to be dispensed as a suppository, unless otherwise directed.

▶ Asian patients may ask which foods to avoid, when taking a medication.

▶ Doctors from different nations also have an exaggerated belief in certain diseases:

- The English believe in virus infections.
- Americans believe in food allergies.
- French believe in liver insufficiency.
- Germans (and Asians) in cardiac insufficiency and low blood pressure.

Dietary customs

Some ethnic diets may affect the course or the treatment of a disease. For example, karela (an Indian vegetable), onion and garlic have hypoglycaemic effects. Karela curry is becoming an increasingly popular dish in Britain especially among those who frequent local Indian restaurants. Karela can not only lower blood sugar but also potentiate the action of insulin or oral hypoglycaemics, which can induce a prolonged state of hypoglycaemia. A hakim, a muslim alternative medicine practitioner, may prescribe this for a diabetic patient. Unbeknown to both the hakim and the doctor, an Asian patient may be using medication from both practitioners and even eating a karela curry at home.

Religious conviction

Religion is a particular system of faith and worship in which a follower believes in and worships a superhuman controlling power, especially a God or gods. It has a controlling influence on a person's everyday life. There are six major religions in the world and it is prudent that a doctor or nurse shows respect for a patient's religious beliefs whatever their own convictions (Boxes 11.4 and 11.5). This is required by the Patient's Charter 1992.

Box 11.4. Followers worldwide (1992).	
Christianity	1833 million
Islam	1026 million
Judaism	18 million
Hinduism	733 million
Buddhism	315 million
Sikhism	18 million

Info. 95, Helicon (1994)

Box 11.5.

'Of course it is right that people should hold their beliefs and their faiths strongly and sincerely, but perhaps we should also have the humility to accept that, while we each have the right to our own convictions, others have a right to theirs too.'

Her Majesty The Queen
1987 Christmas Broadcast

Science and religion

Apparently, science and religion have contradictory thinking (Box 11.6) and there have been many open conflicts between the two in the last millennium. They now join hands in patient care particularly in holistic medicine and palliative care. Many health professionals, managers and patients now try to benefit from both disciplines by involving local religious leaders in solving religious conflicts in a patient's treatment whenever such a need arises. A question about religion is likely to be included in the British Census 2001. Under the Race Relations Act 1976, Jews and Sikhs are considered as religious as well as racial groups.

Box 11.6.

Science	Religion
Objectivity and reason	Subjectivity and intuition
Approach:	Approach:
Practical	Theoretical
Analytical	Empirical
Critical	Moral
Unemotional	Emotional

Spiritual pain

A devout religious person may experience a feeling of intense guilt, fear and worthlessness when he or she has broken a religious taboo, e.g. eating cow's meat for a Hindu or eating pork for a Muslim or a Jew. A similar feeling can occur in patients after eating products of these animals. Spiritual pain can be accompanied by nausea, vomiting, distress and can occasionally turn into anger against him/herself or others. It should be recognised as a clinical entity.

Spiritual pain may not respond to counselling or behaviour therapy but may be alleviated by counselling and prayer rituals by a respective religious leader: a priest for Christians, a rabbi for Jews, a maulana or imam for Muslims, a pundit for Hindus, a monk for Buddhists and a Giani for Sikhs (Box 11.10). A practice manager should keep a list of telephone numbers of local religious leaders and contact them when appropriate.

Greetings

Appropriate greetings can give a kick start to a medical consultation or a transcultural contact with colleagues at work.

▶ Christians and liberals from other religions would say 'Hello' or 'Good morning/afternoon'.

▶ Muslims would greet by saying 'Assalam-u-alaikum'.

▶ Jews would say 'Shalom'.

▶ Hindus greet with 'Namastay'.

▶ Sikhs say 'Sat sri akal'.

Three things need to be remembered:

▶ Christians, Jews, Muslims and liberals from other religions would shake hands with a person of the same sex.

▶ Devout Hindus, Sikhs and Buddhist would not shake hands but raise two hands together.

▶ Devout women from all religions would not shake hands. Some liberals might do so.

If a doctor is not sure of the appropriate greeting, just saying 'Hello' or 'Good morning/afternoon' with a smile should be enough. Let the patient offer a hand if he or she chooses (and hope they have not come for the treatment of warts on hands!).

Stycar vision tests

Stycar vision test cards, Toybox and Ladybird books contain pictures of pigs, dogs, dolls and human faces. There are some religious factors which may influence the reliability of these tests.

▶ Jewish and Muslim parents will not keep books with a picture of a pig in the house as the pig is taboo.

▶ Muslims and Hindus from north India consider dogs as untouchable animals and will not encourage their children to talk about them.

▶ Dolls and pictures of human faces are unacceptable to devout Muslims because they mimic God's work of human creation.

▶ Children from Jewish, Muslim or Hindu religions may take longer to recognise and talk about these objects than their Christian peers. An allowance should be made for this in vision or IQ assessment schedules.

Religious issues

A working knowledge of some religious issues would be helpful in prescribing, compliance and meeting practice targets.

▶ Alcohol in medications, orally or locally may be acceptable by liberal or reformed Muslims but not by devout Muslims. It is best to prescribe alternative products for them.

▶ Gelatin capsules are made of bones and skins of animals including pigs and cows. Devout Jews, Muslims, Hindus and vegetarians may not comply but may not tell the doctor out of politeness. It is good practice to prescribe tablets or other forms of the drugs or negotiate if there is no alternative.

▶ Morphine and opium by mouth or by injections is forbidden in Islam and Hinduism. Where these are needed a negotiated approach is more helpful.

▶ Euthanasia is forbidden in all religions.

▶ The sanctity of life doctrine is acceptable to all religions. This can form a basis of negotiation when a forbidden medication has to be given to a devotee, to save life.

▶ Some devout Roman Catholics and followers of the Orthodox Church may regard physical pain as a part of penance and, therefore, may decline to take analgesics.

▶ Some devout followers of many religions, particularly Islam and Hinduism, may believe in the will of Allah or Bhagwan (God). An illness may be considered related to a broken religious taboo and a prayer ritual can result in healing. They believe that God gives the doctor the power to help in healing.

▶ Beef insulin can cause a religious dilemma for devout Hindus. Pork insulin, though permissible to Jews, may be unacceptable for devout Muslims. Both may be a nightmare for vegetarians.

▶ Measles, mumps, influenza and yellow fever vaccines are made in egg or chick medium and would be unacceptable to vegans. Sometimes practice targets may not be met.

▶ Rubella vaccine was first prepared from an aborted foetus. Some devout Catholics and Muslims, due to their anti-abortion stance, would refuse it.

Health promotion advice

Some health promotion advice, prepared with western habits in mind, may not be heeded by devoutly religious groups (Box 11.7). Advice appropriate to the cultural and religious beliefs of the target population will be more cost-effective.

Box 11.7. Coronary heart disease – prevention and religions.

Do not smoke. But
▶ Sikhism forbids smoking already.
Drink tea, grape juice (red), wine (red) but
▶ Islam forbids alcohol.
Eat oily fish (e.g. sardines) but
▶ Vegetarianism forbids fish.
▶ Judaism and Islam forbid shell-fish (e.g. prawns).

Ethnic distinctions

Ethnic variations or racial characteristics are an important factor in medical science because everyone is born with a unique genetic and ethnic biological make-up. This section is based on my evidence-based research and I have quoted important references accordingly.

Applied anatomy and physiology

Some ethnic or racial distinctions have clinical and medico-legal significance, as follows:

The retina

This is pink in Europeans but chocolate brown among black people and any colour in between among Asians and Chinese, corresponding to their skin pigmentation. Melanin pigment is present not only in the skin but also in the choroid and deep layers of the retina. It protects the lens from developing a cataract due to heat from sunlight, which is more intense in tropical countries. In clinical practice the following points should be borne in mind:

▶ In child health clinics, it is customary to look for the red reflex, to exclude a cataract, by using an ophthalmoscope set on plus 3 and held at 25–30cm distance. Ophthalmoscopy is not easy in black babies whose retina is more heavily pigmented. Do not try to see fundi: it is almost impossible to get an adequate view in a black infant without dilating the pupil (Hall *et al* 1999). There will be a red reflex in white but a grey reflex in black and dark-skinned Asian babies.

▶ As this information is not included in all standard textbooks, it is essential that care be taken in the fundoscopic examination of non-Europeans for assessing the stages of retinopathy in hypertension and diabetes and in diagnosis of retinitis pigmentosa. Although pigmentation of the retina is a normal feature among blacks, a black person may also present with retinitis pigmentosa.

▶ Dark-skinned people are less likely to develop cataracts due to heat, encountered in occupations such as brick making, than their white colleagues. This factor may have an implication in employment and also in compensation claims for occupational damage.

The skin

Melanin pigmentation of the skin has the following clinical and medicolegal implications:

▶ The assessment of pallor, yellowness and cyanosis would be almost impossible in black skin. Therefore, it is more reliable to examine the colour of the mucous membranes of the mouth and conjunctiva, and also the colour of the creases of the palms, when examining black people and dark-skinned Asians. Anaemia is a feature of the colour of the blood and not of the patient and the colour of the skin may be misleading (Swash 1995).

▶ Melanin pigment in the skin has two protective functions when exposed to sunshine, particularly in the tropics.

    – It reduces the incidence of melanomas and skin cancer. However, it should be remembered that the black skin also becomes darker, albeit to a lesser degree than white skin. Nevertheless, skin cancer incidence is greater in whites.

    – It protects photosensitive nutrients, such as folic acid in the blood, from photolysis when exposed to sunlight. Consequently, the normal values of folic acid would vary among whites and blacks.

▶ The colour of a bruise in white and black skins is a medicolegal trap. In whites, a rash is red (erythema) and a bruise is bluish purple (violet) or pale purple (mauve). In blacks, a rash is violet and a bruise is deep dark purple. In a case where an African-Caribbean mother sued an English consultant paediatrician for compensation, I gave evidence to this fact in the Family Division of the High Court, in London. The black child had leg ulcers and swollen wrists due to sickle cell disease, and also had a rash due to allergic dermatitis. The rash was mistaken for bruises and a non-accidental injury was diagnosed. The black parents suffered a lot of distress when they were interviewed by social workers and interrogated by the police.

Clinical medicine

White blood cell count

Evidence from Europe and Africa suggests that black people have a lower range of white blood cells, particularly neutrophils, than whites and other races (McGhee 1993, Adewuyi 1994). According to an American study, the difference is almost 50% (Box 11.8A) (Shaper *et al* 1972). In the UK, some hospital haematology departments, particularly those in mixed ethnic areas, now use separate haematological value scales for white and black patients because some studies (Box 11.8B) revealed unexplained leucopenia among black patients (Shaper *et al* 1972). Familial or ethnic neutropenia was also found in Yemenite Jews because of mixed marriages between caucasians and blacks (Box 11.8C) (Shaper *et al* 1972). The inheritance is by autosomal dominant genes.

This ethnic variation would affect the diagnosis and management of the following conditions:

▶ Leucocytosis occurs in pregnancy (third trimester), malignancy, bacterial infections, myocardial infarction, renal failure, gout, diabetes mellitus, myeloproliferative disorders, post-trauma, post-haemorrhage and as an effect of steroids, beta-agonists, digoxin and lithium.

▶ Leucopenia occurs in viral and bacterial infections, agranulocytosis, folate or vitamin B_{12} deficiency, tuberculosis, typhoid, leukaemia, post-coronary artery bypass graft, serum lupus erythematosis, Felty's syndrome and as an effect of thiouracil, phenylbutazone, mianserin and meprobamate.

Box 11.8A. Total WBC/Neutrophils (American Study: Mississippi).

IN WHITES
    WBC   7,600 mm^3
    Neutrophils 4,560 mm^3

IN BLACKS
    WBC   4,050 mm^3
    Neutrophils 2,025 mm^3

Medicine in a Tropical Environment A. G. Shaper *et al* (eds) London: BMJ Publishers, 1972, pp 322–8

Box 11.8B. WBC (English Study) 'Unexplained Leucopenia in Africans and Caribbeans living in England'.

ONE GROUP

▶ 25 Caribbeans, 5 West Africans and 1 East African:

Neutrophil count   2,210 mm^3
Lymphocyte count 1,670 mm^3

▶ Caribbean children 6 to 24 months tested – they had low neutrophil counts

Medicine in a Tropical Environment A. G. Shaper *et al* (eds) London: BMJ Publishers, 1972, pp 322–8

Box 11.8C. WBC (Israeli Study) 'Familial Neutropenia in Yemenite Jews observed'.

ONE GROUP

A) 62 out of 780 Yemenite Jews (mixed marriages between Caucasians and Blacks) had Neutrophils under 3,000 mm^3 – LEUCOPENIA

B) 33 out of 80 Neutropenic subjects had Eosinophils 350–550 mm^3 – EOSINOPHILIA

Neutropenia and Eosinophilia both transmitted by autosomal dominant gene. Eosinophilia due to helminthiasis was not the whole story.

Medicine in a Tropical Environment A. G. Shaper *et al* (eds) London: BMJ Publishers, 1972, pp 322–8

Box 11.8D. Ethnic haemoglobinopathies.

Afro-Caribbean:	HbC disease Sickle cell disease
Asian (Punjab):	HbD disease
South East Asians/Blacks:	HbE disease
Vietnamese/South East. Asians:	Alpha thalassaemia
Cypriot:	Beta thalassaemia
Chinese:	Prim. idio. acqu. aplastic anaemia

Red blood cells

Haemoglobin, PCVs and red blood cell counts were lower in black infants than caucasian infants and Hbs had no influence on red cell indices (Ogala 1986). The pattern of haemoglobinopathies also differs in various ethnic groups (Box 11.8D).

Pernicious anaemia

This is the most common cause of vitamin B_{12} deficiency in the British white population but is rare in Africans and Asians except in vegetarians (Jenkins 1995).

Of course, any disease can occur in any ethnic group but there are distinct disease patterns in multi-ethnic epidemiology. Differing needs would demand different answers and would have consequences on health care provision and financial resources.

Height and weight charts

Those currently in use in Britain are based on white children from south-east England and 'could be applied' to tall races from Europe, Africa, Asia and America. However, these would not be applicable to normally short races such as the Chinese, South East Asians, Bangladeshis, Sri Lankans, South Indians and Gujaratis. An unwary doctor or health visitor could mistakenly diagnose normally short and lightweight children from short races as suffering from failure to thrive. Some of these children may be on the first or third centile in the growth chart. As the chart fans out with age, the growth may falsely appear to be falling. As there might not be multi-ethnic growth charts available for many years, it is prudent to make clinical judgement allowing for these normal ethnic variations.

Drug response

This also varies with a patient's racial and biological make-up. Acetylator status is the rate at which the body metabolises and inactivates a drug by the acetylation process. Slow metabolisers would retain a drug longer with a better response but also more side-effects. Half the population of the UK and USA are found to be slow metabolisers with 1% of Canadian Eskimos and 82% of Egyptians. More slow acetylators were found in Hindu Indians than in the Chinese and Japanese. Phenalzine, sulphonamides and isoniazid are examples of drugs whose metabolism is found to differ in different races (Whitford 1977). An Eastern person may say, 'Doctor, your medicine was too strong for me, therefore, I took less dosage than you prescribed'. The patient may be a slow acetylator and would need to have a lower dosage. Logically, this variation should affect dosages of all drugs but more research is required.

Cultural encounters in the MRCGP examination

Ethnic and transcultural issues have been asked for in the MRCGP examination for many years but, from May 1998, these issues have become officially a part of the MRCGP examination. As with other core contents, questions in this area may be asked directly or indirectly in all modules (Qureshi 1998). The MRCGP examination changes with time.

Examiners and examinees are all general practitioners from different cultural, religious and ethnic backgrounds. A cultural encounter between them sometimes may be mistakenly attributed to a racial preference. One should take a step back and consider whether a misunderstanding could be a difference in thinking based on different schooling and cultural upbringing.

I have been teaching in MRCGP preparation courses for many years and run tutorials for European doctors about transcultural medicine and for non-British doctors about British examiners and patients. I believe there is a significant culture gap between some examiners and their examinees when they come from different cultures. As with knowledge and skills, this gap can be bridged by education.

The problems in transcultural encounters may fall in the following categories:

Language and colloquialism
The English, Americans, Germans, Asians and Africans speak different types of English language. They also speak at different speeds (Box 11.9).

Box 11.9. Examination communication.

Fast speakers	Slow speakers
Irish	English
Chinese	Indians
Sri-Lankans	Africans

Price of politeness

▶ If a candidate speaks fast and cannot be fully understood, an English examiner may say 'I know what you mean'.

▶ Please speak slowly and clearly making the examiner understand you!

Religious upbringing
Devout followers of any religion, even liberals or seculars, may have a built-in barrier in their training. For example, Muslims or Asian women doctors and patients from different religions might be at a disadvantage in a video-based examination.

Misunderstandings
Limitation of space permits me to quote only five true examples:

▶ A German examinee was annoyed that the English examiner kept asking him about social class issues. Neither were aware that the social class system in Britain is akin to the Hindu (Indian) caste system and this system is not followed by other countries.

▶ A Gurkha candidate kept admiring the examiner's tie and asked questions and lost time in the valuable four minutes allotted for each question.

► An African candidate remained tight-lipped and answered questions in only a few words for fear of saying something wrong. The English examiner tried in vain to find out what the candidate knew.

► A Chinese doctor kept uttering a long list of references, to impress the examiner, in answer to every question. He was annoyed that the examiner would not listen to his list of 20 references.

► A Muslim examinee kept saying 'Insha Allah' (God willing) when the examiner expected the doctor to make his own decision without anyone else's help.

The list is endless but the gap is bridgable by recognising the problem and by mutual social education of both the candidates and the examiners.

Conclusion

The neighbours principle formulated in Donoghue -v- Stevenson 1932 made it clear that the patient is a legal neighbour of the doctor and a duty of care is therefore owed (Scott 1994). There is a growing trend for the doctor–patient relationship to turn into the doctor–plaintiff business. I have highlighted some basic cultural, religious and ethnic factors which should be considered in every medical consultation, in the same way as age, sex and social class has been a part of medical practice. There are many free resources at the GP's disposal (Box 11.10). In a multi-ethnic practice, it is prudent to serve the whole population and deal with every individual patient's needs in an appropriate sensitive way with a caring attitude. This chapter can be used as a starting point; primary care teams should devise their own policy to monitor the quality of care. It should be remembered that clinical medicine, particularly in general practice, is practised beyond textbooks.

Box 11.10. Resources available.

Local

► Priest/rabbi/imam/pundit/giani

► Racial equality council

► Interpreter/linkperson/relative

► MP/Councillor/leader/friend

National

► Commission for racial equality

► Appropriate embassy/DoH

► Voluntary organisations

References

Adewuyi J (1994). African Neutropaenia. *Central African Journal of Medicine* **40**: 108–110.

Hall D, Hill P, Elliman D (1999). *The Child Surveillance Handbook*, 2nd edn. Abingdon: Radcliffe Medical Press, p. 139.

Jenkins G (1995). The blood. In: Swash M (ed.). *Hutchinson's Clinical Methods*, 13th edn. London: W.B. Saunders, p. 412.

McGhee M (1993). *A Guide to Laboratory Investigations*, 2nd edn. Oxford: Radcliffe Press, pp. 13–17.

Ogala W N (1986). Haemoglobin and ethnicity. *Annals of Tropical Paediatrics* **6**: 63–66.

Qureshi B (1994). *Transcultural Medicine*, 2nd edn. Reading: Petroc.

Qureshi B (1998). Cultural criteria in the MRCGP Examination. *British Journal of General Practice*. **48**: 1105.

Scott W (1994). *The General Practitioner and the Law of Negligence*. Chartridge: Business & Medical Publications, p. 8.

Shaper A G (1972). In: Medicine in a tropical environment. London: BMJ Publishers, 332.

Swash M (1995). *Doctor and patient*. In: Swash (ed.). *Hutchinson's Clinical Methods*, 13th edn. London: W.B. Saunders, p. 18.

Whitford G M (1977). Acetylator status and antidepressants. In: *Documenta Geigy – Proceedings of an International Congress on Transcultural Psychiatry*. Macclesfield: Geigy Pharmaceuticals, p. 8.

▶12

Introduction to the Royal College of General Practitioners and its Examination

John J Ferguson

In 1948 at the inception of the National Health Service general practice was a cottage industry with low morale. Nobody had stuffed general practitioner's mouths with gold. Remuneration was by capitation and so the more the doctors spent on their practice the less they would earn for themselves.

In spite of this unpromising start, there was a small band of enthusiasts that felt that things could only get better. The enthusiasts persuaded the Royal Society of Medicine to form a section of General Practice, with G F Abercrombie as the first section President in 1950. This established general practice as a clinical speciality and was a major achievement for the future. It is interesting to note that it was the same band of enthusiasts that, while they worked together at the Royal Society of Medicine, went on to found the College of General Practitioners in 1953, later to become a Royal College in 1967. At the time there was a debate about whether it should be the College of General Practice in line with other colleges or whether it should be the College of General Practitioners. But as general practice is about personal doctoring it was decided that the title should reflect this fact.

G F Abercrombie became chairman of the Foundation Council of the College of General Practitioners. The vice-chairman, Fraser Rose, laid the foundations of the examination as we know it today, and is remembered in the Fraser Rose Medal, awarded to the candidate gaining the highest marks in the MRCGP examination. My contact with the Foundation Council is through my two mentors in general practice: Dr John Henderson, who taught me the value of scientific precision in clinical medicine, and Professor Richard Scott, the first Professor of General Practice in the world.

The motto of the college '*Cum Scientia Caritas*', can be translated as 'With science and with caring'. Jack Norell in his Pickles Lecture in 1984 debated the two parts of this motto and decided that both parts were necessary to describe the work of a general practitioner. So was this the first mention of evidence-based medicine in general practice?

Initially membership was by application from experienced general practitioners and soon the college had a foundation membership of over 6000 doctors. However, from then on in, membership would only be by examination and in 1965 the first examination was held on 'clinical medicine in the setting of general practice'. Five candidates sat the examination and four passed, giving a pass rate of 80%. Though the pass rate has varied a bit over the years that approximates to the present situation achieved by young doctors at the end of vocational training. Over the first decade or so it was only a minority of general practitioners that sat the membership examination and it is only since 1985 that the majority of young doctors completing vocational training has sat the examination.

The format of the examination has changed over the years. There were three written papers: a multiple choice question paper, testing knowledge appropriate to general practice; a modified essay question paper, pioneered by the RCGP, to test the problem-solving skills with patients; and a traditional essay question paper. There were then two orals, the first one on the practice and your patients and the second on questions of the examiners' choosing.

Examinations can drive the agenda for change. In the 1980s there was much exhortation for young doctors to read, which largely fell on deaf ears. Under my chairmanship the critical reading paper was introduced and, following that, young doctors started reading as if it was going out of fashion! To ensure broad professional competence, which cannot be tested within the MRCGP examination, candidates have to provide evidence of proficiency in cardiopulmonary resuscitation (CPR) and in child health surveillance (CHS). They also have to demonstrate their consulting skills by video assessment or, if that is not possible, by simulated surgery assessment.

Over the years the exam has developed to make it more reliable, repeatable and relevant. The traditional essay question paper has been abolished and replaced by the critical reading paper, and now has been merged with the modified essay question paper to form Paper 1. The multiple choice question paper has developed, and is now Paper 2. The content of the orals has formalised and is planned using a grid to ensure that all relevant areas are covered in the course of the two orals, The examination continues to evolve and candidates are therefore advised to contact the College for a copy of the current regulations well in advance of their application (contact at the end of this chapter).

So why do doctors want to take the MRCGP examination? Richard Wakeford's study in 1989 showed that it was for three reasons. Firstly to demonstrate that the candidate was as good as his or her peers, secondly that it would help them to become a trainer in the future and, thirdly, it would help them to become a Principal in general practice. Today my guess is that the first two reasons still apply, but the third is probably less relevant with fewer young doctors training for general practice and with more vacancies on offer. The expectation that most young doctors would sit the exam at the end of vocational training has not yet been achieved due to the uncertainty over the summative assessment arrangements and the modular format of the current MRCGP examination. However, the MRCGP increasingly becomes seen as a quality marker in general practice.

Most British general practitioners are likely to become members by examination. Under my chairmanship I was charged with looking at implementing membership and fellowship of the College by assessment. Fellowship by assessment has now been implemented, but membership by assessment, for those doctors unable to demonstrate their competence by examination, has yet to be implemented.

Most MRCGP candidates attend some form of preparation course. I was on an RCGP advanced course in general practice in 1972 and met an army officer, Ken Young, on that course who was trying to find out more about NHS general practice, and how Service doctors could prepare themselves better for the MRCGP examination. He went on to found the famous 'Millbank' series of week-long preparation courses aimed primarily for Service doctors but also open to non-service doctors. With the assistance of these courses the pass rate for Service doctors approached that of those coming out of the best vocational training schemes. When the Triservice Department of General Practice left London for Gosport, it was recognised that a void would be left in London. John Richardson, the Military Professor of General Practice, hoped that the Royal Society of Medicine would take over the running of the Millbank course in London for non-military doctors, which it has now done. The content of this course, and this book, follow very much the pattern laid down by the Millbank course to help people understand the format of the examination, and how to prepare for it, and to identify key subjects likely to be helpful in the examination.

Many MRCGP preparation books have been written over the years. The original was *The MRCGP Examination: A Comprehensive Guide to Preparation and Passing* by Ken Young, Tommy Bouchier-Hayes and Alistair Moulds in 1978. Its publication served to demystify the examination and Jack Norell, the then Dean of Studies at the RCGP, said that this book detailing the format of the exam and how to prepare for it meant that 'the MRCGP examination would never ever be the same again'.

Further Reading

Godlee F (1991). MRCGP: examining the exam. *British Medical Journal* **303**: 235–238.

Lancet (1990). Editorial: Examining the Royal College's examinations. *Lancet* **335**: 443.

Royal College of General Practitioners (1990). *Examination for Membership of the Royal College of General Practitioners (MRCGP). Occasional Paper 46.* London: RCGP.

Tombleson P, Wakeford R (1989). Why do trainees take the membership examination? *Journal of the Royal College of General Practitioners,* **39**: 168–171.

MRCGP Enquiries

Examination Department
The Royal College of General Practitioners
14 Princes Gate
Hyde Park
London
SW7 1PU

Phone: 0207 581 3232
Fax: 0207 225 3047 or 0207 584 3165
email: exams@rcgp.org.uk

Information and news about the examination that may be of interest to candidates is posted periodically on the College's Internet website: http://www.rcgp.org.uk

►13

Paper 1

Margaret Murray

The written paper

The written paper (Paper 1) is one of the four modules of the MRCGP examination. It is a marriage of two former papers: the MEQ (modified essay question) and the CRQ (critical reading question). It first appeared in the May diet of the examination in June 1998.

It consists of 12 questions to be answered in 3 hours and 30 minutes. This includes 30 minutes to read the presented material which accompanies some of the questions.

The written paper is set by a nuclear group with input from all members of the panel of examiners and an educational consultant.

What does the written paper test?

It tests anything relevant to British General Practice (Moore 1998), a large and complex area that frequently changes! The Royal College of General Practitioners publishes a series of information sheets about General Practice, including one on *The Structure of the National Health Service* (RCGP Information Services).

The Panel of Examiners collectively devised a blueprint of the domains of competence, for the whole examination (Neighbour 1998):

A. Factual knowledge.
B. Evolving knowledge: uncertainty, 'hot topics', qualitative research.
C. The evidence base of practice: knowledge of literature, quantitative research.
D. Critical appraisal skills: interpretation of literature, principles of statistics.
E. Application of knowledge: justification, prioritising, audit.
F. Problem solving: general applications.
G. Problem solving: case specific, clinical management.
H. Personal care: matching principles to individual patients.
I. Written communication.
J. Verbal communication: the consultation process.
K. The practice context 'team issues', practice management, business skills.
L. The regulatory framework of practice.
M. The wider context medico-political, legal and societal issues.

N.   Ethnic and transcultural issues.
O.   Values and attitudes: ethics, integrity, consistency, caritas.
P.   Self-awareness: insight, reflective learning 'the doctor as person'.
Q.   Commitment to maintaining standards: personal and professional growth, continuing medical education.

Paper 1 examines A–E, G–I, (J) K, M, N and (P). There can be overlap and flexibility. J is also examined in the consulting skills and oral modules. P is also examined in the oral module. The domains can be tested in a variety of contexts.(Neighbour 1998) The doctor as:

Clinician	Employer
Family physician	Manager
Patient's advocate	Business-person
Gatekeeper	Learner
Resource allocator	Teacher
Handler of information	Reflective Practitioner
Team member	Researcher
Team leader	Policy-maker
Partner	Member of a profession
Colleague	Person and individual

What skills the written paper actually tests have been analysed by studying candidate responses (factor analysis) to the written paper (Munro 2000). These are:

▶   Informed decision making /problem solving/clinical management.

▶   Evidence based practice.

▶   Critical appraisal.

▶   Challenges/dilemmas/consequences.

▶   Values/sensitivity/empathy.

Preparation

'The best preparation for the written paper and indeed the whole examination is to get as much experience as possible in all aspects of general practice. Reflecting on one's work, particularly clinical work is an important part of the learning process.' (Figure 13.1)

It is human nature to leave examination preparation to the last minute, but an early start can pay dividends.

Many candidates find it helpful to set up a study group. This helps motivation and prevents isolation. Members can research different topics and critically appraise papers for presentation and discussion within the group. This approach can also help

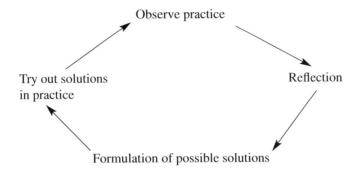

Figure 13.1. Educational cycle (after Kolb).

in preparation for the Oral Module. It is more useful to have a 'topic'-based approach than to read through whole journals at a time. It is not necessary to learn exact references. The contents of the paper, the issues it raises and how they might affect the way you practise are more important.

The Royal College of General Practitioners does not publish a reading list, but useful journals would include: the *British Medical Journal*, the *British Journal of General Practice* and *Evidence-Based Medicine*.

General practice journals such as *The Practitioner* and *Update* publish 'Symposia' taking an in-depth look at different clinical subjects. *The Practitioner*'s series 'How I treat ...' is a useful series of articles which look at a different clinical or ethical problem in practice. You can compare your approach to the problem with that of the authors, usually two general practitioners and a consultant.

Read publications such as the General Medical Council's *Duties of a Doctor*, *Drugs and Therapeutics Bulletin*, the MERC bulletin from The National Prescribing Centre, *Effectiveness Matters* (from the NHS Centre for Reviews and Dissemination, The University of York).

The explosion of information technology is having a huge impact on doctors as well as patients. Sixty percent of Internet searches are said to be health related. Many journals are available on-line as well as in a written format. The Cochrane (2000) Collaboration of randomised controlled trials is available on compact disc. Bandolier (2000) is another useful evidence-based health care journal.

As well as clinical issues, it is important to keep up to date with 'hot topics' and current events in medicine.

There is a list of suggested reading at the end of the chapter. Do not forget the classic literature of general practice (RCGP 1999/2000).

When preparing for the examination, make sure that the information is up to date. The modular examination started in May 1998. The college produces its regulations for the examination on an annual basis and this includes a past written paper. Available on the college website http://www.rcgp.org.uk. The marking schedules are not published.

Types of question in the written paper

Questions designed to test your knowledge and interpretation of GP literature

These (RCGP 2000) usually take the form of: discuss or evaluate the current views of a topic with regard to the evidence on which it is based. There may also be questions about how this evidence will affect or change your current clinical practice.

Working in a group can certainly help in the 'paper work'; it can also help identify common clinical topics. Collecting papers that are relevant to everyday clinical problems is more useful than the random reading of journals. What are the controversies? Learning references is not necessary, it is more important to know the contents of a paper and how the evidence has contributed to the management of a condition.

Papers published in the the *British Medical Journal* now include a table: 'What is already known about this; What this paper adds'. As well as papers do not forget books, systematic reviews, meta-analyses, RCGP occasional papers and national guidelines. The librarian at your local postgraduate medical centre may be able to help you in a literature search.

Example

Upper respiratory tract infections: How does the evidence help you treat patients who ask for antibiotics ?

A: Sarah, 19, a student who has had a sore throat for 24 hours

B: Peter, 33, a telephone engineer who has had sinusitis for 3 days

---

A: The majority of sore throats are viral (approximately 70%). There is not a quick way of finding out if viral or bacterial. Swabs may indicate carriage of an organism rather than acute infection. A sore throat has usually resolved itself in a week. Antibiotics can reduce the duration by about half a day. Prescribing for viral infections adds to the problem of antibiotic resistance; large numbers of patients would have to be treated to prevent the rare complications of sore throats – quinsy, nephritis or rheumatic fever.

The evidence comes from:

▶ a summary in the *MeReC Bulletin* (National Prescribing Centre) Volume 10, number 11, 1999.

▶ DelMar CB, Glasziiou PP (1998). Antibiotics for the symptoms and complications of sore throat (Cochrane Review). In: The Cochrane Library, Issue 3. Oxford: update Software.

B: Sinusitis. Diagnosis can be difficult and is usually made on clinical grounds in general practice. The definitive test at the moment is a CT scan of the sinuses. In one study 85% of patients improved after 10 days without antibiotics. If an antibiotic is used the drug of choice is amoxycillin.

The evidence comes from a meta-analysis:

▶ Brown GG (1998). Antibiotics for acute sinusitis in general practice. *British Medical Journal* **317**: 632–637.

There are complications from antibiotic treatment for whatever it is prescribed: rashes diarrhoea and candida. Drug interactions, particularly with the oral contraceptive pill, have to be considered and appropriate advice given.

Questions that test your ability to evaluate and interpret written material

The written material may be an extract or a summary of the methods and results from a published paper. Audits and drug company literature have also been used. These questions test your critical appraisal skills.

Critical appraisal – a quick summary

▶ The research question – is it relevant to your practice?

▶ The study design – is it appropriate?

▶ Methodology–randomised controlled trial, numbers, bias.

▶ Main outcome measures and presentation of results.

▶ Conclusions – are they justified.

Statistics
Candidates are expected to have a knowledge of simple statistical ideas:

Confidence intervals	Intention to treat
P value	Bias
NNT numbers needed to treat	Odds ratio
Relative risk	Absolute risk
Different types of trials	Positive predictive value
Sensitivity	Specificity

Example

One of your partners states at a practice meeting that he thinks routine peak flow records are of no use in monitoring asthma.

How would you respond, basing your answer only on the critical appraisal of the study below?

Do asthmatic patients correctly record home spirometry measurements?

Asthma diary cards for entering measurements of peak expiratory flow and subjective symptom scores are widely used in clinical trials[1] and have been recommended for guiding management.[2] We compared the record keeping of peak expiratory flow and spirometry measurements of two groups of patients with asthma, with only one group knowing that all data, including time and date, were being electronically recorded and stored by the spirometers.

Patients, methods and results

We recruited 33 adults with asthma (16 men; mean age 52 (range 19–78); mean peak expiratory flow before use of bronchodilator 58% predicted (35–117%)) from the chest clinic of Guy's Hospital. All patients were receiving inhaled steroids and β_2 sympathomimetic agents.

Patients randomly received either a hand-held spirometer (with, unknown to the patient, electronic recording and storage) plus conventional diary card or a combined electronic spirometer and diary card.[3] Patients were asked to record peak expiratory flow, forced expiratory volume in one second, and forced vital capacity twice daily at prearranged times for eight weeks. The electronic diary card spirometers incorporated an alarm, which reminded patients to take the measurements; we suggested to the patients with conventional diary cards that they could use an alarm clock as a prompt.

Patients with conventional diary cards copied the results displayed on their spirometers into their diaries by hand. Patients with electronic diary card spirometers were told that their data were being recorded electronically and did not keep a written record of results. Six of the 16 patients with conventional diary cards and one of the 17 patients with electronic diaries withdrew from the study in the first week (six because of lack of time, one because of admission to hospital). The remaining 26 patients completed the study. We compared entries on the conventional diary cards with the data held electronically to identify incorrect manual entries.

The table shows the proportion of entries for which no corresponding data were recorded with the spirometer (invented entries) and the proportion of entries made more than six hours after or before the correct time (mistimed entries). Completed entries (as a proportion of the expected total) and the accuracy of timing were significantly greater in the patients with electronic diary cards than in those with conventional cards ($P < 0.05$ and $P < 0.001$ respectively; Mann–Whitney U-test).

Incorrect entries on conventional asthma diary cards and accuracy of timing in recording peak expiratory flow and spirometry in 26 subjects with conventional or electronic diary cards.

	Conventional diary card (n=10)			Electronic diary card (n=16)		
	Mean	Median	Interquartile range	Mean	Median	Interquartile range
Completed entries as % of expected total	70	61	58–92	86	94	64–100
% of entries that were incorrect						
Invented*	4	1	0–8	NA	NA	NA
Mistimed+	22	10	1–38	NA	NA	NA
Invented or mistimed	26	14	2–38	NA	NA	NA
Maximum error in timing(h)‡	5.6	5.4	5–8	1.7	1.9	1 to 2

*Entries for which no corresponding data were recorded with spirometer
+Entries made more than 6 hours after or before the correct time
‡Excluding entries mistimed by more than 12 hours

The candidate should consider the methodology of the paper. Firstly its strengths: it is an important problem, relevant to everyday practice. It is a prospective cohort intervention study. The sample has been randomised

The candidate should also consider the weaknesses of the study. The patients had a wide age range. The sample size was very small. There were no records of how the patients were randomised, or of details of any training given to them for meters or diary use. The hand-held meters did not have an alarm and the electronic meters did not have manual recording.

The results
Both groups had a wide similar interquartile range of percentages. There is a wide discrepancy between the median and the mean for 'mistimed' and 'invented or mistimed' categories – which suggests that only a small number of participants are very poor at recording, leading to a biased result.

(The mean is the average, the centre of a normal distribution curve. The median is useful for a skewed distribution curve. It is the mid point value. The interquartile range is a measure of dispersion represented by the difference between the first and third quartiles of a sample. It contains 50% of the observations.)

In some patients there is poor recording of home peak flow readings. This appears to be due to a small number of 'rogue' patients only. One possible explanation is older patients (study to age 78) and no reminder alarm system. This study was carried out in a hospital chest clinic; further studies are needed, preferably in a general practice setting.

Questions that examine your ability to integrate and apply theoretical knowledge and professional values within the setting of primary health care in the UK

These questions cover everyday general practice: the patient, the primary health care team, practice management as well as ethical and medico political issues. How would a competent and sensitive general practitioner deal with these issues? Also look at the issues from the patient's point of view.

These questions test your ability to:

▶ Demonstrate skills in problem solving, prioritising and decision making in a wide range of clinical settings.

▶ Display insight into the psychological processes affecting the patient, the doctor and the relationship between them.

▶ Recognise the family, social, occupational, environmental and cultural contexts of ill health.

▶ Demonstrate communication and consultation skills.

▶ Understand the principles of preventive medicine and the promotion of good health.

▶ Demonstrate appropriate use of resources, including drugs, treatment facilities, referral agencies, other members of the health care team, ancillary staff and complementary practitioners.

▶ Show familiarity with the general practitioner's role in practice organisation, administration and management.

▶ Appreciate ethical principles and the general practitioner's terms of service.

▶ Be aware of current or foreseeable trends and developments in primary care.

Example

Melissa, a 19-year-old, on your list asks you to prescribe methadone for her.

What factors would you consider before giving her your reply?

The first factor to consider would be the patient herself, her past medical and psychiatric history. Are you aware of any drug addictions? Why is she asking for methadone at this time? Is she trying to come off heroin or other drugs? Is she already getting methadone from elsewhere? Is it for her or does she plan to sell it on? What are her social circumstances? Do you feel threatened by her?

The doctor would need to consider his own feelings and experience of prescribing methadone. Has the patient been referred, to a consultant in substance abuse or to a community team? He may want to consult with his partners, and the practice team. Is there a practice, or a local policy on the management of drug addiction? Has the patient been notified to the Regional Drugs Database?

He would need to consider the conflicting pressures on him to prescribe. The Government and Health Authorities would like GPs to take on more of this work. GPs are not so keen, especially after arrests of doctors, when patients have died after taking methadone prescribed by them.

Example

What makes a practice team successful?

The candidate would need to consider the goals of the team, both long and short term. Are the team goals realistic? How are they achieved and monitored? Is everyone working towards the same goal? Issues such as the leadership of the team should be considered, as well as the team dynamics. What are the team types and personalities? (See Belbin's work on management teams and Myers Briggs' work on personality types.) Does the team have any team building exercises such as 'Away Days'? How does it make decisions?

Communication is very important for all teams, the larger the team the more difficult it becomes. Failure of communication is the basis of many patient complaints. The team should have regular meetings, informal as well as formal, to facilitate communication.

Questions in new format

Some of the types of question that have been piloted in the past now appear regularly, e.g. short structured answers. Controversial clinical topics may be listed. The page is divided: on one side you are asked to list the controversies; on the other, to comment on them, with any evidence to support your statements.

The panel can set a question two weeks before the written papers are taken. This allows recent developments to be tested. A last-minute question was set in May of 1997 after the General Election. Candidates were asked to consider advice that they could give to the new Minister of Health. Change continues in the NHS and the latest developments can be treated as oral questions as well as in the written paper.

Any new ideas, from the panel!

The last question of the written paper has often been different, either in format, (extended matching questions first appeared here) or in content.

Good preparation as well as lateral thinking helps in answering this type of question. Do not panic it is the same for everyone!

How is the written paper marked?

Each question is marked by a different group of examiners, led by a cell captain. The whole group has an input into the construction and testing of the marking schedule for their question. The third type of question in the written paper is marked by looking at the constructs of the question. The constructs are the main themes of the question; they are a tool to help the examiners award marks. Full marks can be obtained by giving the best answer possible, under examination conditions. If one of the main themes of the question is not discussed then no marks can be given. Try to think beyond the purely clinical aspects of a question.

How to do well!

Examinations, no matter how well you have prepared yourself, are stressful! Take time to read the instructions and the questions *carefully*. At every diet of the examination candidates lose marks by answering a different question from the one that has been asked.

The written paper is in a combined question and answer book. Each question is on a separate page, with any extra written material required. Each question is marked by a different group of examiners, so avoid cross references to previous answers.

Attempt all of the questions and write legibly. The examiners try very hard to read bad handwriting, but sometimes it is impossible; short notes are acceptable. Try to think as broadly as possible about the question and the issues that it raises.

If you feel 'stuck' over a question, think 'real life'. Has a situation like this arisen in your practice? What were the dilemmas and the issues? How did you, or another member of the team deal with it?

At the start of the question, some candidates find it useful to jot down lists such as 'ideas, concerns and expectations' 'physical, psychological and social' 'doctor, patient practice', etc. Do not be restricted by them, as they could discourage lateral thinking. Quoting every jargon phrase that you have ever come across will not gain marks.

'Should I go on a course?' is a question frequently asked by examination candidates. A course can never substitute for reading, or for experience gained in practice. It can however be useful to meet other candidates, particularly if you are not able to join a self-help group. Courses that include practice for the oral component of the examination can be particularly useful.

Preparation courses are run by a variety of organisations. The Royal College of General Practitioners runs an examination preparation course. Information can be obtained from the Courses Unit. Some of the College faculties run courses themselves; contact your local Faculty Office for details, or your local Director of Post Graduate General Practice. The Royal Society of Medicine in London also runs an annual course.

The skills learned preparing for the written paper will be useful for a future career as a clinician and life-long learner in General Practice. With revalidation imminent they will not have too much time to atrophy!

Good Luck!

References

Bandolier (2000). Internet publications *http://www.ebando.com*

Belbin R, Meredith R. *Management Teams, Why They Succeed or Fail*? Butterworth-Heinemann.

The Cochrane Collaboration (2000). Update software *http://www.cochrane.co.uk*

Kolb D (1984) Experiential learning: experience as the source of learning and development. Englewood Cliffs, NJ: Prentice-Hall.

Munro N *et al* (2000). Exploration by factor analysis of candidate response patterns to Paper 1 of the MRCGP Examination. *Medical Education* **34**: 35–41.

Neighbour R (1998). The modular MRCGP examination in context. In: Moore R. *The MRCGP Examination*, 3rd edn. London: RCGP, Ch 3.

Moore R (1998). *The MRCGP Examination. A Guide for Candidates and Teachers*, 3rd edn. London: Royal College of General Practitioners.

Myers–Briggs (?) Type Indicator, Oxford Psychologists Press

Quenk, Naomi L. Essentials of Myers–Briggs Type Indicator Assessment, John Wiley and Sons.

RCGP Information Services. London: RCGP.

RCGP (1999/2000). Publications Catalogue. Available from the Royal College of General Practitioners.

RCGP (2000). Examination for Membership Regulations. http://www.rcgp.org.uk

Further reading

Clarke R, Croft P. *Critical Reading for the Reflective Practitioner, A Guide for Primary Care*.

Clinical Evidence – a compendium of the best available evidence for effective health care, published biannually by the BMJ Publishing Group.

Essex B. *Doctors' Decisions and Dilemmas*. London: BMJ Publications.

Greenhalgh T (1997). *How to Read a Paper*: The Basics of Evidence-based Medicine. London: BMJ Publications.

Hauff D. *How to Lie with Statistics*. Harmondsworth: Penguin.

Ridsdale L. *Evidence-based General Practice*. Philadelphia: W.B. Saunders.

Neighbour R (1998). *The Inner Consultation*. Dordrecht: Kluwer.

Tate P (1997). *The Doctor's Communication Handbook*. Oxford: Radcliffe.

Acknowledgements

The following are thanked for help and advice from Dr Davis Haslam, Chairman of the Examination board of Council of the RCGP. Dr Andrew Wilson, the written paper Convenor. Dr Neil Munro and Dr John Sandars, members of the written paper nuclear group. Dr Clare Searle, my partner.

▶14

Paper 2

Tim Swanwick

In the beginning was the multiple choice paper. Answers to multiple choice questions were usually selected from a list of five and were frequently guessable just from the structure of the question. Guessable that is if you were not put off by negative marking, a system which intimidated those of little confidence and tempted the foolhardy. A multiple choice paper would test isolated and often arcane bytes of knowledge and repeated sittings, even of the same paper, rarely produced an improvement in performance due to the uncontextualised nature of the information at stake.

As you would expect, the MRCGP examination's machine-marked paper has moved on considerably and is now a sophisticated assessment tool of high validity and reliability. It incorporates a variety of question formats testing not only knowledge but also a deeper understanding of that knowledge and its application to day-to-day general practice.

Content

The MRCGP examination has a masterplan or blueprint dictating the areas of competence that each component should test. This is why it is quite easy to pass three modules and fail a fourth – or vice versa!

Paper 2 sets out to test the following areas:

▶ Core factual knowledge.

▶ Emerging knowledge.

▶ Application of knowledge.

▶ Critical appraisal.

The distribution of marked items among these areas changes year-on-year, but currently around 15% of marks are allocated to critical appraisal and the remainder distributed equally between the other three areas.

Core factual knowledge is the bread and butter of general practice: the diagnosis of migraine, regulations surrounding prescription writing and so on.

Emerging knowledge refers to information that has entered the arena of general practice within the 18 months prior to you sitting the examination.

Application of knowledge is about your problem-solving skills and your ability to select a solution based on the best information currently available.

In testing these domains of competence the paper will ask questions on general medicine, surgery and medical specialities, e.g. dermatology, ophthalmology, ENT, women's health, child health and service management.

Critical appraisal questions will test your ability to interpret data. You will need to have a basic understanding of the commonly used statistical terms including those used in evidence-based medicine, e.g. calculation of number needed to treat (NNT). Calculators will not be needed and so are not permitted in the examination.

Format

The paper comes in two sections. Section 2 comprises what remains of traditional multiple choice questions. In these multiple true/false questions a statement is followed by a variable number of items, any, all or none of which may be correct:

Example 14.1.   Multiple true/false question.

In the examination of the eye:

1. Cyclopentolate drops can be used to dilate the pupil.

2. The green light on an opthalmoscope is used better to visualise lens opacities.

3. Near vision of N5 is better than N1.

4. A substantial minority of males are colour blind.

5. A bilateral visual acuity of 6/60 qualifies for blind registration.

Section 1 is full of more inventive and adventurous formats and, examiners being the people they are, this section is being gradually expanded at the expense of Section 2. For example in 1998 there were around 350 true/false items and 50 items in novel formats. In May 2000 there were 180 and 120 items in each section respectively.

This shift reflects the examiners' increasing interest in testing the application of knowledge as well as their exploration of ways of assessing critical appraisal skills following the demise of the Critical Reading Paper. The drop in the total number of items is necessary because of the increased time it takes to read through a Section 1 question.

So what are these novel formats? There are four main types in current use but watch this space, the examination does not stay still for long.

▶   Single best answer (SBA).

▶   Multiple best answer (MBA).

▶   Extended matching questions (EMQ).

▶   Summary completion questions (SCQ).

Single best answer

A statement or stem is followed by a variable number of items only one of which is correct. That is to say it is the best response out of a list of possible options:

Example 14.2.   Single best answer question.

A 54-year-old man is being treated for hypercholesterolaemia discovered after a MI 6 months ago. He has been taking simvastatin 10 mg at night for the last 2 months. He had a fasting lipid profile and LFTs checked by the practice nurse a week ago and attends to discuss the results which are as follows:

Total cholesterol   4.7 mmol/l

LDL cholesterol   3.2 mmol/l

HDL cholesterol   1.05 mmol/l

Bilirubin   5 (normal range 1–17)

ALP   98 (normal range 98–382)

AST   80 (normal range 5–35)

Choose from the following list of options the single most appropriate management option at this consultation:

A   Increase simvastatin to 20 mg at night

B   Change to pravastatin 10 mg at night

C   Change to bezafibrate 400 mg at night

D   Stop simvastatin

E   Continue simvastatin 10 mg at night

F   Change to atorvastatin 20 mg at night

Multiple best answer

A statement is followed by a variable number of items, a specified number of which are correct:

Example 14.3. Multiple best answer question.

A 65-year-old smoker presents with a gradual onset of breathlessness on moderate exertion, and a cough with clear sputum. Chest examination reveals general reduction of breath sounds and the presence of a few rhonchi bilaterally. Spirometry reveals an FEV1 of 50% of that predicted. Identify the three most appropriate therapeutic interventions to be considered following the British Thoracic Society COPD guidelines 1997.

A   Salbutamol inhaler

B   Beclomethasone inhaler

C   Ipratropium inhaler

D   Salmeterol inhaler

E   Sodium cromoglycate inhaler

F   Oral theophylline

G   Oral steroid trial

H   Nebulised ipratropium

I   Referral for long-term oxygen therapy

Extended matching questions

A scenario has to be matched to a list of options. There may be several answers that appear likely but you must choose only the *most* likely from the list.

Summary completion questions

These are difficult questions to write and so are kept closely guarded under lock and key. A summary of a given piece of written material is presented which has had various key words deleted. Your task is to fill in the gaps from a list of terms supplied.

Validity, relevance, clarity and discrimination

Paper 2 is designed to test knowledge relevant to general practice. It is set by a group of general practitioners and the pass mark is likewise determined by general practitioners. You will not be tested on irrelevancies. Each question has been carefully selected to test what it declares itself to test as clearly and unambiguously as possible. In the pursuit of clarity an entire lexicon of terminology has been developed. These terms will be reproduced in the introduction of your exam paper so you do not have to memorise them.

Example 14.4. Extended matching question.

Theme: Chest pain

Options:

A Angina pectoris	H Mitral stenosis
B Aortic stenosis	I Musculoskeletal chest pain
C Compression fracture of spine	J Myocardial infarction
D Dissecting aneurysm	K Pericarditis
E Herpes zoster	L Pneumonia
F Hyperventilation	M Pneumothorax
G Oesophageal spasms	N Pulmonary embolism

For each patient below select the most likely diagnosis. Each option may be used once, more than once or not at all.

1. A 55-year-old business man who ruptured his right Achilles tendon one month previously has his leg in a plaster of Paris cylinder. He complains of progressive shortness of breath and chest pain worse on taking a deep breath.

2. A 20-year-old shop assistant complains that she cannot get her breath, that her chest feels tight and her fingers are numb. Her peak flow is normal and her chest is clear. You note that she is breathing rapidly.

3. A 78-year-old man after a head cold became short of breath and developed a cough productive of yellow sputum. He is pyrexial and you note areas of diminished breath sounds with fine crepitations at the right base.

4. A 55-year-old man presents with sudden onset of crushing central chest pain at 4.00 am. He is vomiting and sweating, very frightened and his blood pressure is 100/55.

5. An 80-year-old woman lives in sheltered accommodation. She has had falls with loss of consciousness from which she makes a quick recovery. She admits to chest pain on exertion and of feeling giddy. She has a basal systolic murmur radiating to the neck.

6. A 19-year-old student has sudden onset pain in the left side of his chest. He is very short of breath and is slightly cyanosed. His left lung is resonant with absent breath sounds.

Finally, questions are designed to be discriminating. In short this means that some will seem easy and some will not!

And the marks

▶ All items count to your final score.

▶ There is no negative marking.

```
┌─────────────────────────────────────────────────────────────────────────┐
│ Example 14.5.   Terminology.                                              │
├─────────────────────────────────────────────────────────────────────────┤
│ A particular feature is:                                                  │
│                                                                           │
│ characteristic, pathognomic, diagnostic, occurs in the vast majority      │
│ typical, significant, common                                              │
│                                                                           │
│ when it is found in at least 60% of cases                                 │
│                                                                           │
│ in the majority                                                           │
│                                                                           │
│ when it occurs in more than 50% of cases                                  │
│                                                                           │
│ in the minority                                                           │
│                                                                           │
│ when it occurs in less than 50% of cases                                  │
│                                                                           │
│ low chance, in a substantial minority                                     │
│                                                                           │
│ when it occurs in up to 30% of cases                                      │
│                                                                           │
│ has been shown, recognised, reported                                      │
│                                                                           │
│ when found in authoritative published evidence. No implication is         │
│ intended about the frequency of occurrence.                               │
└─────────────────────────────────────────────────────────────────────────┘
```

▶ The pass rate for this paper was 78.4% in October 1999.

▶ A pass in Paper 2 gains approved exemption from the summative assessment multiple choice paper.

▶ The top 25% of candidates in Paper 2 are awarded merit.

Preparation

Prepare early.

Treat every patient you see as a potential learning experience. Ask yourself in the consultation, 'Do I really know enough about this condition?' and 'Am I offering the best modern management?' Reflect on each patient contact and jot down in a notebook those things that you need to know. If you really *need* to know something it will stick much better when you eventually find out. Do not leave it too long though as we all tend to patch over those uncomfortable holes in our knowledge rather quickly.

Avoid indiscriminate reading of journals or text books. There are many more reasons to write a paper than there are to read one! Target what you need to know as a general practitioner, and in the main stick to high quality review articles, meta-analyses and consensus statements. Questions are derived principally from the *British Medical Journal* although it would be well worth looking at the following:

- *British Medical Journal.*

- *British Journal of General Practice.*

- *Drug and Therapeutics Bulletin, Adverse Drug Reaction Bulletin.*

- *Evidence-Based Medicine, Clinical Evidence.*

- Bandolier, Effectiveness Matters, London: DoH.

Courses are useful, especially those looking at critical appraisal skills.

Small groups meeting regularly are a good way painlessly to review the latest literature. Remember that some of the questions relate to current best practice and should be answered in relation to published evidence. This may differ from local arrangements.

Practice papers are available but do not necessarily reflect this season's look. They are useful for self assessment purposes and a sample paper can be obtained from the RCGP sales office. A set of floppy discs, the Phased Evaluation Programme (PEP), can be ordered from the RCGP in Edinburgh.

On the day

Arrive early. Read the lozenge filling instructions carefully. Answer all the questions – you have nothing to lose. You can mark the question paper but leave time at the end to transfer your answers to the Opscan sheet. Remember to leave the question paper behind, failure to do so might result in disqualification. Above all, do not panic, you know more than you think you do.

Further reading

Sample Paper 2 (without answers) available from The Sales Office, RCGP, 14 Princes Gate, London SW7 1PU.
Phased Evaluation Programme discs available from PEP Office, RCGP, 12 Queen Street, Edinburgh EH2 1JE.
Godlee F (ed.) (1999). *Clinical Evidence*. London: BMJ Publishing.
Greenhalgh T (1997). *How to Read a Paper. The Basics of Evidence-based Medicine*. London: BMJ Publishing.
Moore R (ed.) (1998). *The MRCGP Examination. A Guide for Candidates and Teachers*, 3rd edn. London: RCGP.

►15

The Consultation

Richard Styles

Importance

It would be easy to forget that the consultation is pivotal to our work in primary care; whilst we have many responsibilities for organising, planning and gate-keeping healthcare in the UK, it is within the consultation that we should be able to bring our skills to fruition by delivering effective patient care.

Because of our historical pattern of consulting – defined morning and evening surgeries – and our other functions as GPs we find ourselves consulting at a speed unmatched by our European colleagues. It is therefore even more important that we use our time effectively. A 10-minute consultation is the ideal but many doctors see patients at 7-minute intervals and some of this time is taken up with interruptions and logistics.

In this chapter I bring together a range of differing perspectives so that the reader can develop a truly eclectic vision of the consultation to enhance his or her style. There is of course no correct way to consult and we should be wary of structures that are too rigid and inhibit our natural and varying communication skills; rather we should use these viewpoints to enhance our own styles of consulting to deliver a natural but effective product.

Not only is the consultation pivotal to primary care and our training geared towards performing some 8000 consultations in a year, but an understanding of the consultation also gives us an insight into the doctor–patient relationship which enhances our professional lives and helps us to guard against the stresses of our profession. Furthermore, The Panel of Examiners recognises good consulting as one of the prime attributes of a successful candidate.

Effective consultation

A truly successful consultation is like a great picture. You can analyse and appreciate some of the individual components. But it is the overall seamless and skilful construction of these individual parts producing a much greater whole that marks the skill of the consultation.

Most patients will consult their doctors some three to five times per year. This rate is dependent upon demographic features such as age and sex (women, children and the elderly have a higher consultation rate), social class, the availability of other healthcare professionals such as nurse practitioners and also on the doctor's behaviour. Some doctors have high recall rates and some make their patients over-dependent. Some of this consulting takes place in the setting of family medicine where there are many serial consultations but an increasing proportion of our mobile population see their doctor as a one-off fix for an individual problem and we need to be increasingly sensitive to this viewpoint.

To consult effectively in 10 minutes or less we must have a clear view of the dynamics surrounding a consultation and how we can use our time flexibly and effectively. But first can we define what a consultation is? Byrne and Long (1976) refrained from doing so and we may be best served by taking a broad view that a consultation is a social exchange in which a patient seeks some form of health-related advice, treatment or opinion from a medical practitioner. This embraces all the occasions when we are really unclear why the patient is sitting next to us and perhaps we should ask, 'What is it you want me to do?'

Spence (1972) suggested and defined the structural and dynamic points of the consultation such as giving the patient time, listening and being receptive to clues, giving strength and comfort. He considered that consultations should be mutually beneficial and that they are often recognised by both doctors and patients as highly meaningful and defining social exchanges.

It would be tempting to think of the consultation as a static social exchange rather like the confessional but nothing could be further from the truth. Many external factors affect the consultation such as patient awareness, prescribing budgets, gate keeping, evidence-based medicine, advocacy and nurse practitioners to name but a few. These external factors can change quite rapidly as we redefine the delivery of healthcare in the UK.

Pre-consulting

Before we examine the consultation it is worth thinking about what patients do before they come to their doctors and this is often referred to as pre-consulting behaviour. Historically many patients talked to mothers or grandmothers or the local chemist and checked out symptoms with a nurse or health visitor but in our changing society there is increasing dependency upon books and magazines, the Internet and such new agencies as NHS Direct. There is also evidence that patients plan their use of time within the consultation and are mindful of the pressures under which doctor's work. To this extent they may arrive with well-structured opening remarks and lists of symptoms.

Equally the good doctor prepares for the consultation by reading the notes, familiarising himself with current problems, hospitalisation and treatment and thinking about how he may approach the forthcoming interchange. Such preparation nearly always leads to a polished consulting style that makes effective use of time and increases the patient's confidence.

We will now look at many of the different schools of thought that influence the way we consult. It is for the reader to choose those that he feels are important but the ability to recognise and use all in some consultations is one of the factors that makes for skilful and effective consulting.

Diagnosis

Historically much of general practice adopted a medical model where diagnosis was of paramount importance. This was and is still a model learnt in hospital years and is a convergent thought process. It was important at the inception of the NHS to make diagnoses because new drugs such as the penicillins had a huge impact on life. We must never forget that good diagnostic skills are still important in delivering emergency care and in diagnosing conditions for which there are effective treatments. Indeed the whole thrust of evidence-based medicine is dependent upon the condition being diagnosed!

However we must accept that we probably make firm diagnosis in less than 50% of our consultations and that the medical model fails to recognise that much of the illness that we see is caused by social factors such as marital breakdown, conflict, stress at home and work, failure and loneliness. How many of our patients are affected by these conditions and how many outcomes are dependent upon their resolution or amelioration? The holistic school of thought recognised that illness is closely related to personal experience and that many outside environmental and sociological factors play a part.

Social influences

The medical model often relates to a single consultation but much of our work takes place with serial consultations and some doctors see members of a family over many years so a picture of their social milieu is continually developing.

Sociologist were not slow to point out that both doctors and patients have social norms and health beliefs and, whilst these are lessening in this millennium, they were quite markedly different in the 1950s. Both groups function according to their norms and historically this led to the practice of authoritarian and doctor-centred medicine. Of course social factors also affect the way in which we seek help for illness and its effective outcome. We need only compare the depressed, intelligent, mother in an affluent commuter belt, well supported by her family and peers, with the single mother in a bed sit, who may be unsupported and have poor verbal skills, to appreciate how social factors influence the presentation and outcome of the disease.

Doctors have always held a certain position in society and this is true of nearly all cultures, even those where the role of doctor is not so openly recognised and accredited. We do need to be aware that patients feel that we have a certain authority and sometimes this impinges upon the consultation. Patients feel that we are wise and often ask us questions about new advances and treatments. Perhaps some see in us what is called moral authority – a sense that we have an ethical viewpoint, on many issues such as euthanasia and confidentiality and they will wish to know our views.

Certain patients invest strongly in their doctors; historically such a group has been pregnant women who wish to lay down good relations with the carer of their forthcoming family. It is thought that all patients in nearly all societies recognise their 'doctor' as the broker of death and, despite all the advances in palliative care, there are still times when we bring care and comfort, support and dignity to the dying; patients recognise and expect this for themselves and their families. Death is perhaps a moment of primeval medical practice.

Within many societies people use what is called a folk model for illness. They ask: what has happened? why has it happened to them? why now? what would happen if I do nothing and what should I do about it and whom should I see? I think these thoughts are still very prevalent. Many patients feel that alternative therapies are more suitable for their illnesses and increasingly ask our opinions and recommendations.

Interactions

An understanding of transactional analysis gives us a great insight into the interactions within the consultation. First we must appreciate the three ego states in which we all operate: as parents (dominant, didactic, authoritarian and non-listening); as children (subservient, dependent and not taking responsibility); and as adults (responsible, co-operative, recognising our own skills and those of others, and working in partnership).

Much of family medicine was practised with doctors as parents and patients as children. The doctor, who would often adopt a medical model, would dominate consultations, and patients' health beliefs and autonomy would be ignored. Not surprisingly patients took no responsibility and over a period of years became increasingly dependent upon their doctors who in turn became increasingly tired and stressed.

Occasionally patients are quite dominant, acting in the parent role and, whilst we may feel threatened and usually out of control when faced with this situation, it is often worth sitting back and enjoying being a child. The patient will reveal much of their psychology in a few moments and the doctor will gain a great insight into their personality and how they react with others!

Ideally consultations should operate in an adult–adult theatre where both patient and doctor take responsibility and recognise each other's strengths and skills; diagnoses are often discussed as are treatment options and responsibility for follow up is often handed over to the patient. The consultation leaves both patient and doctor with enhanced self-esteem and cements an equal relationship.

It is worth noting that not all consultations can work in this mode. Some patients find it very difficult to adopt an adult culture and those that are very ill or scared are often happy to hand over to the doctor. We should reflect how much we should allow people to be dependent when they are truly ill and frightened.

Balint's concepts

Moving away from transactional analysis we should stop and consider the work of Balint a psychologist whose influence was prominent in the 1960s and 1970s. Balint led us to understand the process of somatisation of psychological disease – its presentation with physical symptoms and the psychological sequelae of disease processes especially chronic disease. He recognised that doctors have feelings about patients within the consultation and that we should recognise and use those feelings in a therapeutic way both for ourselves and our patients. He also developed the concept that doctors should be more sensitive to what is in the patient's mind. Indeed one of the great skills of a doctor is the ability to enter the patient's mindset and see the illness from their point of view. Balint coined the phrases 'the doctor as a drug' suggesting that we had a major therapeutic role as doctors, and 'the anonymity of care' a concept by which nobody stopped and tackled the patient's major underlying problems. From an understanding of these principles we have come to recognise the importance of both the doctor's and patient's personality in dealing with an illness.

Health beliefs

Knowledge of patients' health beliefs has become to be recognised as important in good consulting and the question 'What do you think has caused your illness?' allows us a great insight into the patient's thinking and often relates to their own folk model of illness. The acquisition of health beliefs both on the side of doctor and patient is a complex social activity but it greatly affects the way in which we view illness and the way in which interventions can succeed or fail. Our ability to influence health beliefs is of paramount importance in changing patient behaviour and this is often seen in preventative medicine.

Structure and non-structure

Stott and Davis (1979) brought many of these ideas together when they talked about the exceptional potential of the consultation and delineated their four important areas: managing the presenting complaint; modifying health-seeking behaviour; managing continuing problems; and practising opportunistic health promotion. They began to bring together much thought about the structure of the consultation and, coupled with society's flirtation with structuralism in the 1970s, we saw the birth of many structured approaches to the consultation with some very complex rating scales and tools for their assessment. We should be wary of embracing very rigid models of consulting. They are rather like painting by numbers, the result is safe and just passable but rarely inspiring. Rather we should try and encourage individuals to develop an intuitive style that is free of major flaws but is polished and effective.

There has recently been growing debate about the decision making process that we use as doctors and recognition of some of the important but non-logical functions of the right side of our brains. Supposedly they are the areas that sort vast amounts of experience very rapidly and give us the sense that a patient is unwell and needs urgent admission although there is no logical explanation for this. I am sure we all recognise this sixth sense. We should recognise and be happy with the importance of these non-logical processes and their role in determining how we consult – often in a rather non-structured manner!

Roger Neighbour in *The Inner Consultation* has done much to enlighten us about the importance of these mechanisms and to escape from an over structured view. Despite this it is important to recognise several landmarks or signposts within the consultation. I have already talked about pre-consulting behaviour in both doctors and patients and feel I only need reiterate that doctors should undertake it more often!

Procedure

The welcome is always an important part of any consultation and it worth looking at its function. How do you welcome patients? Do you call for them with an electric buzzer or collect them from the waiting room? What is your non-verbal behaviour at this point? Maybe the good welcome says hello, renews an old relationship, says I have time for you, says I am prepared for you, says what is important for you and puts the patient and doctor at ease.

The next signpost is allowing the patient to present the problem. Often this follows the welcome but there is sometimes a period of interchange over a preceding illness or social event – the doctor's or patient's intuition will normally suggest what is appropriate. Most consultations fail because the patient is not given time and space to present their problem; either the doctor does not listen or quickly formulates an hypothesis about the illness and begins checking it out. In many complaints the listening phase seems to have been summarily curtailed by the doctor. Yes the doctor will need to gently elucidate the nature and history of the problem and the patient's health beliefs as well as how it affects them socially – and that means we have to know what job they do! Most of this can be done with a few gentle encouraging questions whilst an interrogative manner will add little information.

At this stage the patient should be feeling that they have space to develop their anxieties and the doctor's manner should be quiet and encouraging. The patient is handed the adult task of mapping out their problems and the doctor listens in an open and attentive way. These dynamics help to enhance the relationship and allow the doctor and patient to 'connect', as Neighbour describes the process. The doctor will then begin to ask some elucidating questions which help him to formulate the nature of the problem. Occasionally a skilled doctor will have a sense of the problem and will ask an open question to allow the patient to expand on their home or work life. Sometimes the doctor will have a sense of the real problem and ask a more closed question such as 'Do you think you're still grieving for your mother?' which may deliver the problem in what is described as the 'flash' – a moment at which the patient and doctor are both accurately aware that the problem is in the open.

Examination is not always appropriate, and is sometimes not expected by the patient. Indeed you may wish to explore the patient's expectations around this area;

but touch can be important in the consultation and can allow the doctor to make the patient feel safe. In British society doctors are an isolated group who are allowed to touch people – the clergy certainly are no longer free to touch – and within a professional context we should be happy to recognise that touch can be important and therapeutic. Equally difficult is humour. Correctly used it can be of help but at times is misunderstood and seen as patronising. The doctor must rely on his own persona and be mindful of his patients' reactions in both these areas.

After the history and examination ideally there should be some shared (or adult) understanding of what the problem is and this should be followed by an explanation of the therapeutic or management options. Depending upon the complexity of the problem, the verbal skills of the patient and the deductive powers of the doctor, this will have taken a shorter or longer time. Hopefully time has been used effectively and little devices like reading the notes before and getting the patients to declare all their problems before serially undressing and redressing are helpful. If the exchange has taken place in an adult–adult way the patient doctor relationship will have been enhanced en route.

At this point younger doctors will feel the pressure of time and will have to quickly make a decision about ongoing chronic problems and opportunistic healthcare. We must also realise that some consultations are complex and that some patients already have information overload and it would detract from the importance of the presenting condition to embark on these secondary issues. If the patient is a serial consulter they can be safely left until another appointment. Perhaps we need to ask is there any vitally important secondary function that must be completed at this point? I would suggest a pragmatic approach to time management and that it is more important to spend time listening to the major complaints in a doctor's early years and to develop this habit than to try and achieve everything in every consultation.

However the patient should leave the consultation with a clear sense of what to expect in the current illness, what they can manage themselves and when they should or can return. Neighbour calls this process 'Safety Netting'. It gives the patient permission to return if all is not well.

Housekeeping

The term 'Housekeeping' refers to the concept of doctors regaining a psychological equilibrium after a complex or emotionally taxing consultation. Probably in no other sphere of life do individuals have to cope so rapidly with such differing emotions as joy, grief, pain and fear. Coping with these emotions can take a heavy toll on us as individuals and occasionally we need to take some time to adjust before the next consultation.

Learning

Every consultation is a potential learning experience and the good doctor should be able to reflect upon a consultation and capitalise on its educational potential. It would be foolhardy to think we could do this for every consultation but general practice offers most of us at least one learning experience every day and we should develop some strategies for using these experiences for our own personal development or for research. Keeping an occasional record of interesting or challenging cases in a log is an excellent idea.

Empathy

Lastly we are left with some special consulting skills that are worth reflecting upon. We have already talked about listening and asking open questions, about touch and humour. The good doctor should be able to be empathetic, and I find there is often misunderstanding between empathy and sympathy. Empathy is the ability to understand and enter imaginatively into another person's feelings; it is maybe the emotional equivalent of entering the 'mind set'. Sympathy is a more objective and detached state in which we are able to share feelings but do not enter into the person's psyche. I think patients are acutely aware of when we are empathetic and these exchanges are very often extremely powerful within the doctor–patient relationship.

Psychology

Much of the medicine we see has a psychological basis and whilst figures vary according to observers probably more than 30% of our work is due to psychological illness. Evidence has shown that we are much more likely to reach a psychological diagnosis when we have time to listen, ask open questions, adopt a relaxed manner and are not confrontational. We should not be afraid of exploring psychological problems when we feel this is appropriate and when we are offered such powerful clues as stress, anxiety, and sleep disturbance or the non-verbal clues of flatness and non-engagement.

Autonomy and advocacy

No discussion of the consultation would be complete without reference to autonomy and advocacy. Autonomy embraces the concept of patients being able to make their own decisions about healthcare and ranges from which doctor they choose to see to whether or not they comply with treatment. We should always try to heighten patient autonomy within the consultation and should be aware that in certain groups of patients, such as those in care in nursing homes, autonomy can be compromised.

Advocacy is the ability to act on the patient's behalf to ensure they receive the best care. It was always considered a prime function of the family doctor but the levelling out of care that is enshrined in primary care groups means that there are pressures on strong advocates to curtail their activities. Despite this, certain disadvantaged groups will benefit from their doctor being an advocate. Of course one of the greatest inequalities in the delivery of primary health care is that vocal and healthy patients who have good knowledge of health issues consume much more consulting time than those with poor health and poor vocal skills. Perhaps our greatest responsibility as advocates is to redress this imbalance.

Children

There are special skills in consulting with children and letting them take a role in decision making from an early age rather than merely listening to their often anxious parents. We should not be afraid to talk to children as adults, sometimes asking their parents to leave the room. Teenagers require reassurance about confidentiality and a non-judgemental attitude to many of their problems, which often include issues of pregnancy, sexuality and substance abuse as well as depressive illness. Consulting with third parties – the patient's wife or mother – is full of hazards for the doctor. It is easy to compromise confidentiality in the process of being sympathetic or seeming to be the family doctor. Equally we should be aware of making judgements and taking sides in consultations where one member is exposing their view of a family dynamic.

Conclusion

In conclusion we should see consulting as learning for life. It will take us many years to be very polished but the young principal or locum who has an insight into the process can begin to practise caring and very effective medicine. Those practitioners who develop such an insight will find their lives will be greatly enriched.

References

Byrne and Long (1976). *Games People Play.*
Neighbour R (1987). *The Inner Consultation.* London: Kluwer.
Spence (1972).
Stott and Davis (1979). The Future GP Learning and Teaching BMJ.

▶16

How to pass the MRCGP video examination

Peter Tate

The video examination is the only module of the examination over which you have control. This means that if you think about it and prepare for it properly you should be able to satisfy the examiners. However the fact remains that it is not that easy; at present the pass rate is three out of four.

When you apply to the College to take the examination you will be sent an up-to-date Workbook. This will contain detailed instructions and explicit criteria that you need to demonstrate; read it carefully and then read it again. If you are a registrar make sure your trainer reads it too.

This assessment is based on the concept of *competency*, meaning that combination of knowledge, skills and attitudes which when applied to a particular situation leads to a given outcome. You might find it helpful to use the analogy of the driving test. The competency 'three point turn' requires you to turn the car to face the opposite direction, using forward and reverse gears, safely, without endangering other road users, nor striking the kerbs or other obstacles. The number of forward/reverse manoeuvres is not precisely specified, nor is there a time limit, but the examiner would expect the whole process to be carried out with a certain smoothness. Clearly many skills are involved (clutch control, road awareness, steering, etc.), but the competency includes them all, but has a specific, recognisable outcome, namely the car pointing the other way.

Similarly, consulting skill competences have been specified that require you to demonstrate, for example, the ability to discover the reasons for a patient's attendance, by eliciting their symptoms, which includes two competences: encouraging the patient to 'spill the beans', and not ignoring cues. We do not specify *how* the patient is to be encouraged to give account of their symptoms: this may be by open questions, by appropriate use of silence, or some other way. Nor do we need to specify how the cues are responded to. We do expect that at least some bits of unsolicited information are picked up by the doctor.

As you can see a competence is a complex skill, the possession of which is demonstrated by achieving the relevant performance criterion. Possession of the competence does not imply that the doctor uses it all the time. However, unless you as a candidate demonstrates the competence in action, we cannot assume you possess it. You must be clear that the examination is looking for what you *can* do.

From your point of view, the examiners wish you to submit a videotape with a range of challenge that clearly demonstrates your current consulting ability. You might find it useful to look on your tape as a *portfolio of competence*, a collection of effective consultations put together over a period of time. It may help you to consider why the MRCGP introduced a consulting component. The intention was to encourage the learning and teaching of skilful doctor–patient consulting. The examination was seen as a spur to encouraging more time to be spent considering communication as a high priority in the armament of future GPs. To do this a clear definition of what the candidate needed to achieve was created.

The tasks of the general practitioner during the consultation are defined as five units:

- Discover the reasons for a patient's attendance.

- Define the clinical problem(s).

- Explain the problem(s) to the patient.

- Address the patient's problem(s).

- Make effective use of the consultation.

Each of these units is subdivided into elements. For example, in unit one, *discover the reasons for the patient's attendance*, there are four elements.

- Elicit the patient's account of the symptom(s) that made him/her turn to the doctor.

- Obtain relevant items of social and occupational circumstances.

- Explore the patient's health understanding.

- Enquire about continuing problems.

The tasks are too broad to be reliably assessed even at this level. There follows an even more specific level called the 'Performance Criteria' (PC). Each element of the definition has one or more performance criteria, e.g. for the unit *Discover the reasons for the patient's attendance* and the element *Elicit the patient's account of the symptoms which made him/her turn to the doctor*, there are two performance criteria:

- The doctor encourages the patient's contribution at appropriate points in the consultation.

- The doctor responds to cues.

The full definition in addition to the five units has 16 elements and 21 performance criteria.

However to help you further understand what is meant by the performance criteria required for pass and merit here is a detailed description of each one required by the current examination.

Detailed guide to the performance criteria

Discover the reasons for a patient's attendance

Elicit the patient's account of the symptom(s) which made him/her turn to the doctor
PC: the doctor encourages the patient's contribution at appropriate points in the consultation.

This PC has the outcome of an adequate account of the presenting problem: it requires you to demonstrate *active* listening skills; you will not achieve it simply because your patient, unprompted, gives a good account, as some do. Active listening means showing evidence of attentiveness, not interrupting, reflecting back answers to create follow-up questions, as in, 'What do you mean by *dizzy*?' There should be evidence that the doctor can encourage a contribution from a patient who needs to be encouraged.

PC: the doctor responds to cues.

A cue is a sign made (whether consciously or not) by the patient, and capable of being perceived by the doctor. Not every consultation contains cues that need a response! However, since responding to cues (about the nature of the problem) is regarded by the examiners as a core competency, it is up you to demonstrate some in your selection of consultations.

Verbal cues may be simply what is said, some may be what is not said and may be related to the tone of voice, facial expression, posture or actions of the patient. An example of a non-verbal cue would be a visibly sad patient, to whom you comment 'you seem rather low'. A verbal cue might be the patient saying 'It's my back again'; if you not only addressed the present episode but also explored the previous ones, you would have responded to the cue.

Reflection can be a response to a cue: the patient might say 'and I've felt low this week', and the doctor reply 'low?' Equally the same cue could be responded to by a later statement by the doctor: 'You mentioned earlier that you felt low: could you expand on that?'

Obtain relevant items of social and occupational circumstances
PC: the doctor elicits appropriate details to place the complaint(s) in a social and psychological context.

It can be argued that every problem has social and psychological elements, yet the failure to explore these is a common cause of failure in this module. Choose a consultation where the patient is not well known to you and where you need to elicit the background information in a natural way.

Occupational may mean the patient's job, but could equally be how they fill their day, and crucially how the complaint (symptom, illness) impacts on this. There may also be the reverse situation in which occupation could be affecting health.

The *psychological* dimension is of most obvious relevance where the patient is experiencing significant emotional distress. If the examiner is content that the context (nature of the problem, and the patient's manner) suggests this is not the case, then 'appropriate details' may not include exploring feelings, and you will demonstrate competence simply by exploring the social and occupational factors.

However, this PC is not simply 'psychological and social', but rather the *appropriate* exploration of these areas, for *relevant* items, given the presenting problem. Asking 'So what do you do for a living?' while the prescription is being printed is unlikely to be an appropriate or a timely exploration.

Explore the patient's health understanding
PC: the doctor takes the patient's health understanding into account.

This is a merit-level PC and is overtly 'patient-centred'.

Remember that it sits in the area of 'discovering the reasons for attendance'. It is most simply addresses by asking, once you have heard the patient's story, 'What do *you* think it could be?' There are few situations where such a question, properly and sensitively asked, is not appropriate. (The obvious exception would be when the patient has already told you, as 'I cut my finger this morning while opening a can of beans'!) In a patient with headaches you may ask, 'You have had these headaches for a few weeks now and I was wondering whether you had any ideas yourself as to what it might be due to?' This invites the patient to discuss their health understanding with the doctor, indicating that the doctor is interested and concerned about the patient's understanding about their symptoms. It is quite likely that an open question such as, 'So how are these headaches affecting you as you look very worried?' might elicit a response that satisfies more than one criterion, such as picking up cues, exploring psychosocial issues or eliciting health understanding.

The element above refers to 'exploring', since you cannot take the patient's health understanding into account until you have discovered what it is. A patient who asks 'Do you think it's an allergy, doctor?' has some understanding or misunderstanding of allergies which could be explored by asking 'What makes you think it might be?' Implicit in this is the belief that patients' ideas are intrinsically valid and valuable in understanding the nature of their problem.

Define the clinical problem(s)

Obtain additional information about symptoms and details of medical history
PC: the doctor obtains sufficient information for no serious condition to be missed.

This is the 'medical safety' PC, which addresses the focused enquiry that commonly occurs during the consultation, not necessarily at a particular stage: it may happen during an examination, or later, during the explanation, or even as an afterthought. It is about taking a history in the degree of detail which is compatible with safety but which takes account of the epidemiological realities of general practice.

The PC requires you to recognise, from what has been said, any potentially serious diagnoses that an average general practitioner should consider. These would typically include suicidal thoughts in a patient with depression, malignancy in a patient with chronic cough, change in bowel habit, dysphagia, or weight loss, and so on. Competence may be demonstrated by asking focused, closed questions, such as 'Have you noticed any blood in the stool (sputum, urine)?' or an appropriate suicide question.

Serious need not mean life-threatening. A child with a cough or otitis media should probably be asked about asthma symptoms, or about their hearing. A person with back ache should, unless it was manifestly trivial, be asked about red flag symptoms.

Essentially this PC looks for medical competence in history-taking. It may legitimately be absent when the presenting complaint is very minor. This is one reason why you are advised not to include many minor problems among your consultations.

Assess the condition of the patient by appropriate physical or mental examination
PC: the doctor chooses an examination which is likely to confirm or disprove hypotheses which could reasonably have been formed, or to address a patient's concern.

This is not about competence in performing the examination, which cannot usually be judged on tape, but about the appropriateness of the examination in relation to the hypothesis. The examiner will be thinking, 'Why has the candidate chosen to do that examination?' Sometimes you may say something to the patient that gives a clue to the hypothesis: 'I am just going to look in your ears to see if there is wax there', but more often the reason has to be inferred from the context.

The element specifies appropriate physical or mental examination, and we allow as mental examination any reasonable attempt at assessing mental state, where appropriate. Exploring suicidal intention would be a necessary part in a depressed patient seen for the first time, but perhaps not at follow-up. Formal examination of thought disorder in a possibly psychotic patient and memory testing in one with possible dementia would be included.

Make a working diagnosis
PC: the doctor appears to make a clinically appropriate working diagnosis.

Your diagnosis may be explicit, and declared to the patient, but more often the examiners will infer it from your explanation and management plan. Please make sure that you enter your working diagnosis in each Consultation Summary Form in the Workbook.

Explain the problem(s) to the patient

Share the findings with the patient
PC: the doctor explains the diagnosis, management and effects of treatment.

All these three things should be explained, although sometimes the effects of treatment (e.g. improve the symptoms) might not need to be stated. There must be evidence of an explanation of the patient's problem. The element states that the findings should be *shared* with the patient. A short explanation may be enough but it must be relevant, understandable and appropriate.

Tailor the explanation to the patient
PC: the doctor explains in language appropriate to the patient.

You should avoid medical jargon and explain in words your patient is likely to understand. Remember that words can have opposed meanings for doctor and patient. A patient whose leg is hurting 'something chronic' probably has an acute rather than a chronic pain. Beware of abbreviations (MSU, ECG). If your patient asks for clarification, it is probably best not to choose that consultation for the examination.

PC: the doctor's explanation takes account of some or all of the patient's elicited beliefs.

Clearly this depends on the health beliefs having been elicited (see above) and so is also a merit PC.

The competence can be identified as a reference back to some idea which was expressed by the patient, and which the doctor is addressing, either to affirm, or to modify, or to refute. Thus 'So your irritable bowel syndrome is very likely to be related to the stress you were telling me about earlier', or 'this rash is called psoriasis, and is caused by overactive cells in the skin, but it is probably not affected by what you eat' (having elicited the belief that the rash was an allergy to certain foods).

This criterion cannot be satisfied without having previously identified the patient's health beliefs and is the most 'patient centred' of all the criteria, as it requires true involvement in the patient's narrative.

Ensure that the explanation is understood and accepted by the patient
PC: the doctor seeks to confirm the patient's understanding.

Having given an explanation, it is appropriate, and effective, to check understanding; so it may be surprising that this is a merit PC. However, most candidates do not check for understanding!

It clearly implies the use of a question, 'Does that make sense?', 'Have I made that clear?', 'tell me what you understand by that?' or 'what does the term angina mean to you?' and a dialogue between the patient and yourself ensuring that the explanation is understood and accepted, would satisfy this PC.

More problematic is the cursory 'Okay?' It depends what happens next. If the patient appears to take this as a check of understanding, by responding, it will probably do, but there is a risk that patients will say 'yes' to such a query, because it is far easier to say yes than no! Many doctors add 'okay' to all their explanations, as a routine, without expecting an answer. The context should determine whether there is a real 'seeking to confirm understanding'.

Address the patient's problem(s)

Choose an appropriate form of management
PC: the doctor's management plan is appropriate for the working diagnosis, reflecting a good understanding of modern accepted medical practice.

This does not depend on the working diagnosis being 'right'. It simply relates the management plan to the working diagnosis, and to 'modern accepted medical practice'. (In the era of evidence-based medicine, we must read that as 'modern accepted and, when possible, evidence-based, medical practice'.)

The standard here is what a consensus of MRCGP examiners would reach, with allowance for alternative approaches. Thus depression can be managed by prescribing antidepressants, by arranging cognitive therapy, by using a problem-solving strategy, or by referral to a specialist resource, or in mild cases, by support and careful follow-up by the GP.

Involve the patient in the management plan to the appropriate extent
PC: the doctor shares management options with the patient.

This is the most 'patient-centred' of the non-merit criteria, and also perhaps the most crucial for you as a candidate, since failure to demonstrate competence in this area has been the single most common cause of failing the module. Since sharing options may not be common behaviour, it becomes an important factor in deciding which consultations to submit.

The extent of sharing will vary according to the context 'to the appropriate extent'. This will depend on the patient, how capable they are of engaging in such involvement, and the problem, what sort of options exist. Thus a retired science teacher with newly diagnosed hypertension might expect (or need) to be involved very substantially in a range of options, from lifestyle modification, through choice of drugs, to frequency and nature of follow-up. On the other hand, a learning disabled teenager with severe tonsillitis might not appreciate a discussion of whether to take penicillin for five or ten days, and a simple consideration of whether to use tablets or liquid would be more appropriate.

Sharing management options might include treatment alternatives, referral options, choices of when or whether to review a patient, whether or when a patient should return to work after a period of illness, but must demonstrate your ability to involve the patient in the options that are available. For example, a patient with tension headache might include a discussion of treatments available, e.g. analgesics, relaxation techniques, referral for stress counselling etc or could involve a discussion of the alternative possibilities for follow-up. Simply.saying 'I am going to refer you to a stress counsellor, is that all right?' is not an example of sharing; for all but the most self-confident patients, this is a statement of your intent and not an invitation to discuss options. However a consultation that contains the words options, choices, or alternatives and involves the patient in a *two way dialogue* should fulfil this criterion.

The underlying idea of this PC is 'shared decision-making', whether about medication, referral, investigations, or time off work.

Make effective use of the consultation

Make efficient use of resources
PC: the doctor's prescribing behaviour is appropriate.

The word 'appropriate' implies a judgement against the examiner's norms and, by extension, the consensus of the panel of examiners in deciding what, in the circumstances of this consultation, would be appropriate prescribing.

Deliberate non-prescribing, particularly of antibiotics, can be 'appropriate behaviour' here, as can advice to purchase over-the-counter medicines. There will be cases, however, where a decision about prescribing does not arise, as where the consultation is about a 'surgical' condition (e.g. a hernia) and the plan is to refer, or where the problem is social (e.g. housing), and the plan is to take some administrative action. The competence is simply not demonstrated in such consultations; but remember that in order to pass, you do not need to demonstrate competence in *all* PCs in all consultations, three out five is the current rule.

Establish a relationship with the patient
PC: the patient and doctor appear to have established a rapport.

This criterion requires evidence of the development of a sympathetic relationship between doctor and patient, being mutually responsive to each others' signals. This is something that develops during the consultation as the doctor shows awareness of the patient's cues, understands what the patient is communicating and ensures that the patient understands and is involved in the care. Examiners judge rapport by both verbal and non-verbal signals.

What do you have to do to pass?

You are expected to submit only seven consultations, none longer than 15 minutes. You must use standard VHS at normal speed.

You can achieve three results in this module fail, pass and 'pass-with-merit'. The examiners examine all seven consultations, but the merit decision is currently taken on the first five. The commonest reason for failing is not demonstrating that you can involve your patients in decision making.

How is your videotape assessed?

Your tape and workbook will be assessed by a group of trained examiners who are, by definition, working general practitioners with several years experience. Each of the seven consultations is watched by a separate examiner, working in isolation. The examiners report their findings to a co-ordinating examiner. If satisfactory evidence of your competence in all pass-level performance criteria has been found on at least four occasions you can be sure that your tape will pass. We understand that not every consultation will give you the scope to demonstrate all the pass PCs to the required level. Moreover, at the discretion of the consulting skills convenor and the convenor of the panel three rather than four demonstrations of competence may suffice for some PCs, but you would be wiser to aim to satisfy each PC four times.

As you can see selection is all. It is probably true that many who do not pass the examination have the ability but have not demonstrated that ability on the submitted tape.

To pass this module you must read about the consultation, think about it and most importantly practice it. You need to observe and record yourself regularly, become familiar with your strengths and work on your weaknesses. You must be clear that the seven consultations you select demonstrate you fulfilling all of the pass criteria at least four times.

You may find the use of the critique sheet helpful to select your seven consultations (Box 16.1).

Box 16.1.   A consultation critique sheet.
What was done well and why? How could it be done better?

Discover the reasons for a patient's attendance.
Encourage the patient's contribution.

Observe and use cues.
Obtain relevant items of social and occupational circumstances.
(M) Explore the patient's health understanding.

Define the clinical problems.
Sufficient information for no serious condition to be missed.
A reasonable examination.
An appropriate working diagnosis.

Explain the problems to the patient.
Explain the diagnosis management and effects of treatment.
Use appropriate language.
(M) Use the patient's health understanding.
(M) Check understanding.

Manage the patient's problem.
Make sure the plan is appropriate for the working diagnosis.

Share the management options.

Effectiveness.
Prescribe appropriately.
Develop and use your relationship.

Key. Four out of seven for all the above. PCs in bold are the most commonly absent. Those in italics are merit.

Further reading

Moore R (2000). *The MRCGP Examination: A Guide for Candidates and Teachers*, 4th edn. London: Royal College of General Practitioners.

Skelton J, Field SJ, Wiskin C, Tate P (1998). *Those Things You Say ... Consulting Skills and the MRCGP Examination. A Video Plus Guide*. Oxford: Radcliffe Medical Press.

Tate P (1997). *The doctor's Communication Handbook*, 2nd edn. Oxford: Radcliffe Medical Press.

Neighbour R (1987). *The Inner Consultation*. London: Kluwer.

Pendleton D, Schofield T, Tate P, Havelock P (1984). *The Consultation: An Approach to Learning and Teaching*, 2nd edn. Oxford: Oxford University Press.

Moreton P (ed.) (1999). *The Very Stuff of General Practice*. Oxford: Radcliffe Medical Press.

McWhinney IR (1997). *A Textbook of Family Medicine*, 2nd edn. Oxford: Oxford University Press.

Acknowledgement

With thanks to Peter Campion.

►17

Simulated Surgery

Tim Ballard

The simulated surgery component of the MRCGP was developed as an alternative to the video component of the exam. It is designed to assess similar consultation skills to those assessed in the video. The simulated surgery is currently held twice a year but in the future it may become more frequent. This module involves the candidate seeing a number of cases during a surgery (currently 12). Role players who are members of the public play the cases; they are not professional actors. Each candidate has a consulting station, which they stay in for the duration of the assessment. Each consultation lasts for 10 minutes and is separated by a 2-minute gap. After the first six consultations there is a 10-minute interval where simple refreshments are provided for the candidates. The exam is designed to be as similar to a normal surgery as possible. Each candidate is given a running order for the surgery and a simple set of clinical records for each consultation. These records are necessarily brief and are normally no longer than one side of A4. There is nothing in these notes to mislead you. Each role player has an examiner who accompanies them and they assess you; your total marks are calculated by the independent judgements of 12 examiners.

Who is eligible to sit this module?

This module is currently available for candidates who have an insuperable difficulty in preparing videotaped records of their consultations. Common reasons that have been accepted so far have been:

► Moral or religious objections.

► Not being in permanent practice.

► Practising in an environment where a significant proportion of consultations are not conducted in English.

Applicants from the Muslim community have most commonly requested the moral or religious exemption. Candidates from Saudi Arabia have so far provided the majority of applications in this group. Doctors working as locum practitioners make up the largest component of the second group. It is understandable that requesting to videotape consultations while working in this capacity may cause difficulties. The third group is available for practitioners who spend a significant amount of time consulting in a language other than English. This includes doctors working in Welsh-speaking areas as well as those practising in communities with a high ethnic minority population.

If you feel that you may qualify to take the simulated surgery you will need to apply, in writing to the Convenor of the panel of examiners, stating your reasons. This letter should accompany your main application to sit the exam. It is a good idea to seek approval for this route of assessment at least 4 weeks before the closing date for the exam that you wish to sit.

What sort of case mix is there in a simulated surgery?

Each simulated surgery is made up of a variety of different cases. The aim is to assess areas of general practice that are either common or, if less common, are important to manage well. A good example of this less common type is the breaking of bad news to patients. While we all hope that this will be an infrequent part of our professional lives, there is no doubt that such a situation needs handling with particular skill and sensitivity.

The age range is wide; so far there have been consultations with patients between the ages of 12 and 76. Children may be represented by consultation with their parents. There is an equal, or almost equal, balance between the sexes. Your skills in telephone consultation and in working with other members of the primary health care team may be assessed.

> Useful tip: so far there has always been a breaking bad news case. You would be well advised to plan for the exam with this in mind.

The role players are not there to lead you astray or to trick you. If an answer is given then there are no situations where they are instructed to change their history with further questioning. Where management is being discussed with a patient an initial reluctance to follow a suggested plan may be open for negotiation.

What are you allowed to examine?

There are no situations in this module which require any intimate examinations of a patient, such as gynaecological, rectal or breast examinations. If you do request to examine a patient because you feel it is appropriate, for example, an abdominal examination, the role player is at liberty to decline. If a role player does decline any form of examination, including measurement of BP, you can assume that it is either not directly relevant or, if you had been able to carry it out, that the findings would have been entirely normal.

What sort of equipment do you need to take with you to the exam?

It is very important to remember that you should attend this exam well equipped. There are not the facilities to supply you with items if you are not well organised. You will need to bring with you the following:

▶ Stethoscope.

▶ Sphygmomanometer.

▶ Auriscope and ophthalmoscope.

▶ Patella hammer.

Tongue depressors are provided.

The only form of written material that you are allowed to use in the exam is a copy of the *British National Formulary* (BNF). You are not *required* to bring one with you but you are strongly advised to do so.

What facilities can you assume that you have access to?

This is an exam set in British general practice, in the context of the service provided by the NHS. You can assume that you have access to services normally available within this setting. For example you can assume that you can refer patients for radiological investigations, but that these facilities will be by appointment at a local hospital. You should not assume that there is an MRI scanner in your practice! You may assume that you have a normal, well-equipped surgery and that you have easy access to other members of the primary health care team, along with facilities such as electrocardiography.

Standard members of the primary health care team that you may assume that you are able to involve include:

▶ Reception staff.

▶ Practice managers.

▶ Practice nurses.

▶ District nurses.

▶ Health visitors.

▶ Attached social workers.

You may also assume that you have a well-stocked library of patient information leaflets that are available at the reception desk following the end of the consultation.

You are also able to refer the patient to colleagues in secondary care where you feel this would be appropriate.

Blank prescription pads and medical certificates are provided. You may make notes while the consultation is underway. These notes do not currently form part of the assessment.

How are you assessed?

Unlike the video component there is a fixed marking schedule specific to each case. Each examiner compares your performance to this. The consulting skills that are assessed fall into one of five possible domains.

▶ Information gathering.

▶ Doctor–patient interaction.

▶ Communication.

▶ Management.

▶ Anticipatory care.

Each case is marked using five individual constructs. Any individual case may be differently weighted for different domains. For example one case may contain two constructs representing doctor–patient interaction but have no marks awarded for pure information gathering.

In the first domain your skills at eliciting a history are examined. There is scope to do this by either taking a formal history or by giving the patient the space and consideration to tell their own narrative. This domain also includes gathering information from physical examination and from the records provided.

The second domain looks at skills related to putting a patient at ease and developing a rapport. It is here that marks are also awarded for eliciting their ideas and concerns and for demonstrating empathy. This includes the use of both verbal and non-verbal skills. Showing respect for a patient's autonomy may also form part of the marking in this domain.

The third domain addresses communication skills. An example of this would be the appropriate explanation of an illness or a planned investigation in a way that the patient can understand. When producing an explanation for patients it is sometimes appropriate to write things down or to make very simple diagrams. Demonstrating an ability to share options with a patient is often assessed here, as are skills involving negotiation.

The fourth domain looks at skills needed to form a safe and effective management plan. These include using appropriate investigations, referral to specialists and prescribing. If you issue a prescription then the choice of drug and the dosage that you prescribe it in may form part of the assessment. Sensible use of time and resources may be examined in this domain.

The fifth and final domain is focused on anticipatory care. This often involves a process of 'safety netting'. In this process plans are made for follow-up, where appropriate involving input from the patient. Appropriate health promotion may form part of this component.

The consultation is a complex social interaction between a patient and a doctor. Any divisions or domains are by their nature artificial and act as a method for explaining the process of the consultation or as an aid to assessing it. There are some features that are common throughout. A doctor who adopts a patient-centred approach to the consultation is more likely to arrive at an understanding of a patient's situation and their associated health beliefs. Being patient centred means adopting an approach that puts the patient's thoughts and concerns at the top of your agenda. Once this is achieved it is easier to explain a problem to a patient in a way they are able to understand, taking into account their health beliefs. Once this understanding is achieved then sharing options and negotiating a plan becomes easier. This then naturally leads on to activity assessed in the fifth domain. Anticipatory care involves two separate but interwoven features. The first is the doctor's understanding of the natural history of a condition or situation, and in particular an appreciation of the risks, either physical or psychological that a patient may encounter following the end of the consultation. The second requires an understanding of a patient's ideas, concerns and expectations. Both of these elements need to be addressed to 'enable' the patient and to help them to face the future.

Useful tip: in addition to finding out why you think a patient has attended always try to find out what the patient's perceptions or fears may be about the situation.

Each construct is marked by the examiner based on a shortened version of the oral marking grades.

- G (good) 5 marks.
- S (satisfactory) 4 marks.
- B (borderline) 3 marks.
- N (not very good) 2 marks.
- P (poor) 1 mark.
- U (unacceptable) 0 marks.
- O (omitted) 0 marks.

How are the pass and merit marks calculated?

When the exam is over the examiners carry out an exercise to set the pass and merit marks. This takes into account the overall performance of candidates. There is not a requirement to pass a certain number of consultations but to perform overall to an acceptable standard. It is likely that in the future there will also be a requirement to perform to a certain overall standard in each domain.

The following is an example of a case that reflects a relatively low challenge situation in General Practice.

Topic of case:	Allergic rhinitis
Suggested name for patient:	Megan Hope
Age:	22
Sex:	Female

Role player briefing

Opening statement: 'I seem to have a blocked and runny nose, doctor'.

Allow the doctor to ask questions about your blocked nose, and find out from your replies that:

▶ It has been getting increasingly worse.

▶ It has been present for about 2 months and is not getting any better.

▶ It started after you moved to a dusty old house.

▶ You have not felt unwell.

▶ You have no cough, hoarseness or headache. You have not taken your temperature.

▶ You have not stopped work/college or stayed in bed.

▶ You have taken some decongestants but they have not helped much.

▶ You had a sore throat, which was treated with penicillin, 6 months ago.

You should expect to have your nose and/or throat examined. If either of these actions is not performed gently, show some discomfort.

The doctor should know from your records that you had severe sinusitis 2 years ago and were ill for 3 weeks. You felt exceptionally unwell. One of your concerns, which you should reveal if the subject is raised, is that this nasal congestion might be sinusitis coming back again.

Another concern is that you are anxious to be well for a special social event in 4 days time (e.g. bridesmaid at a family wedding). You would not normally have come for a blocked nose, but hope that treating it will clear it up before the wedding. This concern should be voiced if the doctor prompts for it in any way (e.g. 'Why have you come now?' or 'Is there anything else that worries you about it?').

You are expecting to receive antibiotics, but will be content to receive an explanation as to why they are not necessary. If offered a prescription for antibiotics you will accept it. If asked, you are not allergic to any antibiotics. If the diagnosis of allergic rhinitis is made then you want to know: allergic to what? what can be done to find out? what can be done to treat it? If you are offered a choice between taking an antihistamine or using a nasal spray ask for an explanation of the pros and cons. Make your choice depending on the explanation.

Simulated Surgery	
RECORDS	
Name	Megan Hope
Age	22
Sex:	Female
2 years ago	Severe sinusitis Rx Doxycycline
	Off work – 3 weeks
6 months ago	Sore throat – Rx Penicillin V

Acknowledgements
With special thanks to Dr. Peter Burrows.

Figure 17.1. An examiner's mark sheet.

NAME: Megan Hope		EXAMINER:
EXAM CASE:	STATION:	CANDIDATE NO:

1. Information gathering – Interview/history taking

Good	i) Clarifies history of blocked nose, duration, etc.
	ii) Establishes patient's self management up to now
	iii) Recognises past history of severe sinusitis

Unsatisfactory   History achieves none of the above

2. Information gathering – Physical examination

Good	i) Views nose efficiently without causing discomfort
	ii) Views throat efficiently without causing gagging or discomfort
	iii) Checks for tenderness over the sinuses with gentle pressure

Unsatisfactory   Candidate omits physical examination

3. Doctor–patient interaction – Patient's concerns

Good	i) Sympathetic attitude, not dismissive of trivial condition, and identifies concern over special event before patient reveals it
	ii) Recognises expectation of antibiotics
	iii) Recognises concern that sinusitis could recur

Unsatisfactory   Candidate ignores patient's concerns

4. Communication – Explanation

Good	i) That this is chronic rhinitis
	ii) Likely to be caused by an allergy not bacteria
	iii) Antibiotics of no help in this situation

Unsatisfactory   No explanation of condition

5. Patient management – Options

Good	i) Option given between antihistamines versus topical preparations
	ii) Pros and cons of above explained
	iii) Options of RAST testing or skin patch testing offered

Unsatisfactory   None of these options offered

g – good	**s – satisfactory**	**b – barely adequate**
n – not very good	**u – unsatisfactory**	**o – omitted**

Seriously deficient performance

►18

Overview of Orals

Mike Thirlwall

Introduction

There has been an oral component to the MRCGP examination since it began. Its purpose and structure have undergone much change through the years. Currently, it is intended to assess candidates' decision-making skills – their professional judgement. Questions are frequently found on dilemmas in practice, which are then explored in a series of further questions designed to challenge and explore the candidate's approach to practice. The examiners will be looking for pragmatic, consistent decision-making which is based soundly on ethical principles and evidence.

Unlike the other modules of this examination, it is a personal and dynamic encounter with inherent risks of inconsistency, bias, potential for 'stage fright' and misunderstanding. The Panel of Examiners has worked hard with the help of external consultants to reduce such variables to a minimum by structuring the whole exercise and by training the examiners in the skills of conducting oral examinations.

Candidates will have two 20-minute Orals with two pairs of examiners. None of the examiners will have any idea of how the candidate has performed in the other parts of the examination, or how many attempts the candidate has had at taking the oral module. The pair of examiners conducting the second oral will have no idea of how the candidate fared in the first one.

Structure of the Oral examination

At the start of each day's examining session, the four examiners who will be working together for that session plan the two Orals. They use a grid constructed from the three areas of competence that the Oral is focussing on: communication, professional values, and personal and professional growth and in four contexts which are: care of patients, working with colleagues, society and personal responsibility (Table 18.1).

Between them, they will select questions for each 'box', aiming to ask about five topics in each Oral, so that each area and context will be tested at least once. The questions will have been preplanned by each examiner with a marking scale to rate candidates' responses on a nine-point scale from 'dreadful' to 'outstanding' (both rare!), through 'not adequate'/'borderline'/'satisfactory' in the middle range.

After the plan for the oral session has been agreed, the two pairs of examiners go to their separate tables to receive the candidates. Each pair agrees the order in which they

Table 18.1. The Oral grid.

CONTEXTS	Areas		
	Communication	Professional values	Personal and professional growth
Care of patients			
Working with colleagues			
Society			
Personal responsibility			

will ask their five or six topics (alternately) and share with each other the marking scales for their preplanned questions.

It will help to expand on what is meant by each area and context.

Areas

Communication

The principles of verbal and non-verbal communication. Consultation models (you would be well advised to be familiar with at least one of those in common use in teaching about British general practice). Effective information transfer, motivation, empathy, listening.

Professional values

Moral and ethical principles. Patient autonomy. Medico-legal issues. Flexibility and tolerance (of colleagues and patients alike). Implications of styles of practice. The roles of other health professionals. Cultural and social factors.

Personal and professional growth

continuing professional development (of oneself and others), self-appraisal and evaluation, stress awareness and its management. The risk of burnout. Coping with change. The management of change.

Contexts

The care of patients – specifically.
Working with colleagues (in the PHCT and beyond, e.g. secondary care).
Society as a whole – its expectations and the GP's role.
Personal responsibility (for care, decisions and outcomes).

It may help to illustrate these with some of the topics that have featured in recent examinations.

Communication and:

▶ Care of patients   Breaking bad news. Use of consultation models. Communicating with adolescents.

▶ Working with colleagues   Practice meetings. Team building.
A complaint against a colleague.

▶ Society   Communicating with the media. Health promotion.
Teenagers' health.

▶ Personal responsibility   Aggressive patients. Effective consulting.
Heartsink patients.

Professional values and:

▶ Care of patients   Patient autonomy. Terminal care.
Requests for expensive drugs.

▶ Working with colleagues   Sick doctors. Community pharmacists.
Clinical guidelines.

▶ Society   Rationing. Euthanasia. 'Gatekeeper' role.

▶ Personal responsibility   Advance directives. 'Whistle blowing'.
Gifts from patients.

Personal and professional growth and:

▶ Care of patients   Evidence-based medicine. Which patients make you
stressed? Audit.

▶ Working with colleagues   Burnout. Poorly performing colleagues. Away days.

▶ Society   Out of hours arrangements. Quality of care.
Using new drugs.

▶ Personal responsibility   Hazards of general practice. Continuing medical
education. Coping with uncertainty.

Preparing for the orals

Any candidate who takes an intelligent and active interest in their work should be capable of passing the Oral. Although it can be taken at any time, it would be wise to take it after significant experience of working in general practice, certainly towards the end of the year in general practice, if you are a Registrar. The old adage that 'GP's work in the jungle and hospital doctors work in the Zoo' (with A&E departments possibly on the city limits!) still holds true and the approach to many problems will be different from a GP perspective.

There are few clear-cut answers to any of the problems that we face in general practice and thus there will be few right or wrong questions in the Oral; there is no 'College line'. Thus, a question about a visit request for a child with otitis media might seem straightforward enough but might range across the use of the telephone in general practice, parents' health beliefs, evidence base for treatment of OM, changing patients' expectations of care, the role of nurse practitioners, etc. depending on which area and context the question was being asked in.

It will help to keep abreast of editorials in the *BJGP* and *BMJ* as well as opinion pieces in the other popular publications. The GMC *Guidelines on the Duties of a Doctor* will be essential reading. If you can, form a discussion group with others who are sitting the examination and try to put yourself in the examiners' shoes; try designing discriminating questions on topics in some of the areas and contexts – it is not as easy as you might think!

Many candidates attend preparatory courses for the examination. They can be extremely helpful, especially those which offer the experience of sitting a 'mock' Oral – there is nothing like a dry run with nothing to lose to take away the fear of the unknown.

On the day

You will have plenty of advance notice of the date and time of your Oral so think ahead and check that it does not clash with any other major events in the capital cities (the Orals currently begin in Edinburgh – usually the Royal College of Physicians – and then relocate to London at the Royal College of General Practitioners). Allow plenty of time for your journey so that you arrive in as relaxed a state as is possible.

There is no dress code but, as with other important events in life, you may wish to make a good impression, so clean, smart clothes are what most candidates opt for. A small bottle of mineral water to refresh yourself between Orals might be helpful.

When you arrive at the venue, you will be checked in by a member of staff and given a name badge along with a sheet of instructions for the day. You will be told where to wait and where the toilets are.

Shortly before the Oral is due to start, a member of the Examination Panel will come and give you a short welcome and briefing. You will be told which table you will be going to. Do listen carefully and do not wander off without letting a member of staff know where and why.

Great care is taken to avoid candidates being examined by examiners that they may know and examiners check their lists. Despite this – and largely because of the large number of preparatory courses that candidates can attend – you may see a familiar face. If you feel that this might prejudice your Oral you can ask to be examined by a different pair of examiners. You must decide quickly and let the organising staff know immediately.

Quality control and examiner training are taken very seriously. You may therefore see a third person at your table – he or she will be observing the examiners and the examining process and will take no part whatsoever in your Oral or the marking process. You may also see a video camera at your table – this is trained on the examiners – watching them not you! You cannot be identified apart from your voice. The tapes are only viewed by members of the Examination Panel for teaching purposes.

The Oral itself

At the appointed time, you will be shown to the table for your first Oral. The examiners will introduce themselves to you and let you settle before proceeding. Each question will be clearly introduced – if you have misheard or do not understand do seek clarification – then it will be developed with a series of subsidiary questions to search for the desired responses.

The Oral is timed carefully (you will see stopwatches on the tables) so that each topic is explored over about 4 minutes before the other examiner takes over with the next topic. Once the 20 minutes are over, a gong or bell will sound. The examiners will allow you to finish what you are saying (though nothing 'after the gong' is marked) before allowing you to leave the room to await the second oral.

After 5–10 minutes, you will be ushered back into the room to a different table to meet the second pair of examiners who will go through their five or six topics in the same way. At the end of the second 20 minutes, the examination is complete and you are free to go and relax in whatever way you wish!

Most candidates find the pace of the Oral quite stimulating and feel that the time flies by. In the four minutes available the full range of the question will be explored and you will be encouraged to make decisions. You may wonder why so much is packed in to such a short time. If you think back to some of your other vivas or Orals you may recall getting asked about a topic about which you have little or no knowledge and have then spent a deeply discomfiting 20–30 minutes wriggling under interrogation! The MRCGP Oral is designed to sample as widely as possible to avoid this problem. None of us knows everything and, just as in the written parts of the examination, you are answering a series of questions – each of which will be marked individually before the examiners award an overall grade for the 20-minute oral. Treat each topic individually. If you do not feel you have done well on a particular topic, try and wipe it from your mind as you move on to the next 4-minute topic – rather like a sportsman not worrying about a poor shot but concentrating on the next. Likewise, as you move from one Oral to the next, you are starting afresh so try and set aside the previous 20 minutes and prepare for the next session.

When both Orals have been completed, the two pairs of examiners will meet to collate the grades they have awarded. In order to pass the Oral you have to achieve an aggregate of greater than four borderline grades. Merits are decided on analysis of the overall results of all those sitting the Oral exam at this session. If you have failed, the examiners will make notes to justify their decision and sometimes suggestions about how the candidate might improve on their performance. These are passed on to the candidates who have failed.

Although you are bound to be nervous, try not to let this overwhelm you. The examiners are all working GPs, most of whom have an educational background with great experience of learning and teaching at undergraduate or postgraduate level. They are not out to trick you – simply to find out how you approach problems and issues, and what decisions and judgements you make about them. The majority of candidates pass the Oral. The MRCGP examination has always been an inclusive assessment, unlike many other postgraduate examinations that are exclusive with low pass rates.

If you are unsuccessful, you have another two attempts, without having to resit those modules that you have passed. In your area, there are almost certainly trainers, course organisers or examiners who will be happy to help and advise before you embark on a further attempt.

Good luck!

▶19

Reading and Preparation for the MRCGP

David Smalley

Introduction

When you sit down to think about how to prepare for the exam, it can seem quite daunting. Where do you start? What do you read? What can you ignore? Can you ignore anything! The subject range appears never-ending, and there does not seem to be a simple curriculum and prospectus.

However, having discussed preparation with many candidates and many examiners, I can assure you that there are effective, stimulating and even fun ways to prepare!

Throughout our working lives as GPs, we are constantly working in a changing environment. This provides for an interesting (if occasionally stressful) life – but seldom dull. We need to develop skills in self-assessment, and be able effectively to keep up to date, using techniques of adult learning.

Learning to work effectively for the MRCGP carries almost no disadvantages – perhaps just the time commitment. The advantages are numerous:

▶ Improved knowledge base.

▶ Greater consideration of the depth and range of problems presented to the GP.

▶ Improved self-confidence.

▶ A tendency for more reflective work.

▶ Improved ability to think rationally and broadly about presented problems.

▶ Hopefully, a greater pride in our branch of the profession.

▶ Stimulation to continue learning throughout your career.

The examination is well respected throughout the world, and is eminently achievable for the vast majority of candidates. Convinced yet? … let me continue.

What is being tested?

Consider the following extracts from *The Regulations for the MRCGP Examination*:

'The discipline of general practice has few fixed boundaries, being defined as much by what patients elect to present to us as by our own views on the GP's job description.'

'the Membership examination has no strictly defined curriculum. It sets out to test all those areas of professional knowledge, skills and values which reflect the consensus view of what comprises good practice in the British National Health Service today.'

In an attempt to describe the many generalisable skills, attributes and competencies that make up a good GP, the examination has devised a 'Blueprint' (Box 19.1).

This, perhaps, makes a start in defining the areas to be covered in preparation.

It seems, and is, a big list but it does give you an idea of the range of material that can be covered. Nothing should then come as a big surprise.

The subject of examination preparation becomes even more achievable when you consider the structure of the examination.

Box 19.1. Blueprint.

Domains – generalisable skills, attributes, competencies

▶ Factual knowledge.

▶ Evolving knowledge: uncertainty, 'hot topics', qualitative research.

▶ Evidence base of general practice; quantitative research.

▶ Critical appraisal skills.

▶ Application of knowledge.

▶ Problem solving: general.

▶ Problem solving: case-specific.

▶ Personal care.

▶ Written communication.

▶ Verbal communication: consultation process.

▶ Practice context: management, business.

▶ Regulatory framework of practice.

▶ Wider context: medico-political.

▶ Ethnic and transcultural issues.

▶ Ethics, values and attitudes, *caritas.*

▶ Self-awareness: 'the doctor as person'.

▶ Personal and professional growth: CME, standards.

The modular structure of the examination

Details of the four individual modules are described previously in this book.

Consideration of what each module is trying to test, is the key to effective preparation.

Paper 1 – the written paper

(3 hours and 30 minutes reading time)

This paper tests knowledge and interpretation of general practice literature. It tests your ability to evaluate and interpret written material presented to you, and also examines your ability to integrate and apply theoretical knowledge and professional values.

Its origins stem from an amalgamation of previous MEQ and CRQ elements but there is now a policy of blurring this previous distinction. Each question should be answered in its own right, giving evidence where appropriate.

In this paper will be some questions on 'hot topics'. These are important subjects that have been very prominent in the medical press in the previous 18 months – and they can usually be spotted. If you get a group of about five candidates to try and list together important hot topics, they usually start to slow down after identifying about 20 items. However, they almost invariably manage to pick out the majority of subjects that the examiners have also identified as important, topical and with a sound literature base. This is time well spent as these topics may well be also mentioned in the oral exam, be part of the MCQ, and, of course, your patients will expect you to be knowledgeable about these very same topics.

It is also very worthwhile to practice previous questions. There is a skill factor in being able to identify the separate constructs of the question. It is helpful to practice thinking laterally and broadly. Like any other examination you ever take, it is more important to try to develop a reasonable breadth of ability, rather than to have an advanced but very narrow knowledge base. The first few marks of each question are much easier to get than the last few. This is not surprising when you consider that the marking cribs are developed by a group of examiners sharing and pooling their ideal answers. Unless you have a brain the size of a planet, you are unlikely to get every point mentioned by the examiners (although, if you do mention a relevant point that the examiners forgot, you will get the credit).

Do not panic about giving references if you cannot remember the exact month, authors etc. If you can identify roughly where the paper/book was located and, more importantly, how it supports your answer, you will get credit (but simply saying 'BMJ 1999' will not be enough).

This is also the section of the exam where you will need to be able to demonstrate skills in critical reading and appraisal. These skills were not always taught well (if at all) in medical school, and you may need to practise answering previous interpretation questions. There are several published checklists to help you with this, and you must get familiar and comfortable with one of them, e.g. Box 19.2.

Box 19.2. Critical Appraisal Checklist.

Does the paper address a question relevant to your practice?

Where did the research take place and who are the authors?

Do they have a vested interest?

Design

▶ What type of study; is it appropriate?

▶ Selection of subjects and controls.

▶ Randomised? How was this done?

▶ What were the outcome measures?

▶ Are they clinically relevant?

▶ Are the sample numbers appropriate?

Results

▶ Are all the subjects accounted for?

▶ How are the results presented?

▶ Is the statistical analysis present and appropriate?

Conclusions

▶ Are conclusions reasonable?

▶ Do authors address limitations of the study?

Paper 2 – the MCQ

(3 hours, comprising true/false items and extending matching)

This part of the exam is intended to test your knowledge base. This will include both recent and established knowledge.

Some candidates like MCQs and others find them very threatening; perhaps it all depends on your previous experience. Extensive tests and quality controls are used to make the questions fair, reliable, valid and discriminating. Some of them you will find easy, but several others will be hard. Its supposed to be like that.

Yet again, it makes sense to practise MCQs. There are several published books, and several regions have their own MCQ library. Use this practice to identify lacunae of knowledge, and then do your best to correct them. Reading articles in the popular medical press and standard journals will give you sufficient current knowledge to tackle that aspect of the MCQ.

A few words about technique

There is no negative marking, so have an attempt at everything. Some candidates have found unexpected time difficulties, appearing to be 'caught out' by the extended-matching questions which are usually towards the back of the paper. Although fewer in number than the traditional true/false questions, they do take longer to do. Some candidates elect to do these questions first.

Be careful if you are one of those candidates who write their answers initially on the question paper, and then transcribe them later onto the answer sheet. This is fraught with danger, and certainly makes the invigilators very squeamish.

Consulting skills

(nearly always the 'video' – in certain circumstances, a simulated surgery instead)

Full details of this section are found elsewhere in this book, and in the guidebook issued by the RCGP when you apply to take the examination.

Prepare carefully. Select the cases carefully. You need to present cases which give you a good chance of demonstrating all the required competencies.

Although you now only need seven consultations, they take longer to collect than you think. Remember, you are asked to show that you can demonstrate specified consulting techniques. There is no hidden marking sheet for the examiners. If you do regularly demonstrate the competencies, you must pass.

Orals

The aim of the oral is to explore candidates' decision-making skills. In particular, it looks at the areas of communication, professional values and personal development.

You may well be presented with scenarios or ethical dilemmas that you have not previously experienced. Do not be phased by this; it only reflects our everyday working life. Who knows what particular problem the next patient brings. Experienced GPs continue to see and hear things which are new to them, and long may it be so! What the examiners are looking for is how you approach the problem. There may not be a right or wrong answer, but there is likely to be a range of options, and you are liable to be asked to justify your preferred choice.

You can prepare for this by practising oral exams amongst yourselves. If possible, you can use your trainers, course organisers and possibly a tame local examiner.

I do not think that there is much point in 'hitting the books' for the oral exam. Much more important is being reflective in your everyday work. Also keep an eye on what is topical in the daily newspapers. It is embarrassing if the standard *Guardian* reader knows more than you. Gaining experience in your GP registrar year and discussing dilemmas with your colleagues is probably the best preparation of all.

Before I list favourite journals and books, let me emphasise again the nature of the exam. It is set, marked and validated by everyday working GPs. It looks for a good standard of general practice which should be attainable by GPs. (Admittedly, higher than the 'ankle-high' hurdle that is summative assessment.) It is achievable. It has a high pass rate. There are no catches. Prepare well and you should have few problems.

Examiner survey

Over the last few years, I have conducted an on-going survey amongst examiners about their recommended reading. Although there was a large variety of preferences, a clear pattern emerges of the most useful reading material. There are no surprises!

Nearly all surveyed recommended the following:

▶ *BMJ*.

▶ *JRCGP*.

▶ *Drug and Therapeutics Bulletin*.

▶ *Monitor*.

▶ 'And something about critical appraisal'

These are the most popular recommendations. If you keep abreast of the GP-related articles in these publications for the 12–18 months preceding the exam, you will be very well prepared. You may also find it pleasurable and addictive, which sets you up for the rest of your professional life.

Other journals recommended, but less frequently, were:

▶ *Practitioner*.

▶ *Update*.

▶ *Effective Health Care*.

▶ *Bandolier*.

▶ *MEREC*.

▶ *Pact Reviews*.

▶ Topical items – what is in *The Guardian*.

I think it is important to recognise which journals suit you. It is impossible to read them all, and would probably be counterproductive if you tried.

Numerous books were mentioned, and the commonest are listed in Box 19.3. This list keeps changing, and I think it becomes a personal preference issue. For topical items, the journals are more important.

Finally, from the examiner survey, a few other common thoughts were recorded:

▶ Join/create a study group (Box 19.4).

▶ Practise past questions (but beware of changed exam format).

Box 19.3.   Useful books.

British National Formulary

Balint, *The Doctor, his Patient and the Illness*

Clinical Evidence London: BMJ Publications.

Consultation books, e.g.
Neighbour R (1998). *The Inner Consultation.* Dordrecht: Kluwer
Tate P (1997). *The Doctor's Communication Handbook.* Oxford: Radcliffe Medical Press

Crombie. *Pocket Guide to Critical Appraisal*

Essex B. *Doctors Dilemmas Decisions.* London: BMJ Publications.

Greenhalgh T (1997). *How to Read a Paper: The Basics of Evidence-based Medicine.* London: BMJ Publications.

Oxford series – e.g.
Paediatric Problems in General Practice
Womens' Problems, etc.

Palmer. *Notes for the MRCGP*

Qureshi B (1994). *Transcultural Medicine*, 2nd edn. Reading: Petroc

Sackett. *Evidence-based Medicine*

Box 19.4.   How about a small study group?

▶ Groups of about five reliably produce good model answers.

▶ Share out work of looking for papers on major topics.

▶ All candidates have different strengths and weaknesses.

▶ Reflect on your daily experiences of general practice.

▶ Discuss problem patients.

▶ Look up problems.

▶ Research individual topics. Do not just work through the journals.

▶ Pay particular attention to important topics, and ones where literature has changed practice.

▶ Skills are as important as knowledge, but you need some of both!

▶ Studying is a good habit, and can become enjoyable!

▶ Your time is not being wasted, learning for the exam is also learning general practice.

▶ Group work has a pastoral and supportive role.

▶ Remember major papers on common and important conditions, even if published some time ago.

▶ Take particular note of guidelines of national status.

Summary

▶ Start early and aim to cover wide range of topics.

▶ It may be easier to cover many areas by working in groups

▶ Many of the common and important topics can be spotted and so be the subject of preparation, but . . . while helpful, this will not be enough!

▶ *BMJ* and *JRCGP* over preceding 12–18 months will provide excellent relevant and topical material, but . . .

▶ You will need to identify your own particular areas of weakness, e.g. critical appraisal skills, knowledge of study design, etc.

▶ Practise exam questions/format. Past questions have been published.

▶ Relax! Remember the examiners are all working GPs and mostly human!

▶ Most candidates pass (>70%).
With the modular format, it is 'easier to take, but no easier to pass'.

▶20

Hot Topics

Nigel Holmes

Identification

When making careful assessment of what could be construed as hot topics in the MRCGP, I would recommend that you look at two general areas:

▶ *Perennial hot topics* that regularly come up in the examination, and which have been traditionally, and are expected to remain highly topical for the MRCGP, e.g. British guidelines on asthma management.

▶ *Recent hot topics* that have occurred in the past year or so; these may be short lived, or may themselves become perennial hot topics, e.g. the Viagra issue.

Structuring your learning in identifying and revising hot topics

It is beneficial to set up a small group of like minded MRCGP candidates, ideally 8 months or so before the date of the examinations; about five is an ideal number. Apart from having the obvious goal in working for the MRCGP, you should clearly be able to get on together, and also have the commitment to set aside protected time, at least on a weekly basis, when you can meet in a quiet environment. You may wish to have the same venue for your meetings each time, or locate them around your individual homes or surgeries, but this must be protected time, with no distractions from work, on call, or even family.

Set your goals early, so that each of you has a task of identifying hot topics, and then set about deciding your priorities of which hot topics to revise in detail.

Each member of the group could be allocated a number of different topics to study within a definite time, producing a precis of the hot topic, and a photocopy of references, etc. This is a very time-efficient way of learning, and, in my experience of over 17 years of tutoring candidates, has proved to be very successful.

I shall detail perennial hot topics later, but my recommended and tested method of identifying recent hot topics is to review objectively the *BMJ* and *BJGP* starting with the January issue in the year before the date you sit the examination, i.e. if you sit the examination in May 2001, then study the journals from January 2000 to the current date. Some MRCGP tutors produce lists of articles relevant to the Membership, and I have done this for over 10 years. My personal method is to review the *BMJ* on a weekly basis, and the *BJGP* on a monthly basis, setting aside an hour each Monday evening to scan the journals, picking up articles of general practice relevance. The name of the journal, the date of the article, the name of the article and the author are then recorded on a simple data base on the computer. This could be numbered 1–100 as the year progresses, and then can be easily identified from the computer hard disc. Individual articles can either be read from past editions of the journals, or can be obtained on the Internet (*www.bmj.com*). Be relatively objective in producing such a list; do not just record your own interests.

Prioritising your learning

Having collated a list of GP-orientated articles in the *BMJ* and *BJGP*, the group should then follow this protocol:

▶ Carefully read through the list of articles.

▶ Write down a topic area when it appears, e.g. teenagers, or ischaemic heart disease.

▶ Score against each topic area with a cross each time you see that reference in the list, e.g. if teenage health or articles on teenagers turn up five times, then put five crosses next to that.

▶ Produce a 'top twenty' of topic areas which have come up over and over again, as well as anything innovative or out of the ordinary, e.g. Viagra. The latter, or innovative topics, are often put into the written paper at the last moment, or frequently come up in the oral examinations.

▶ Having identified your top twenty topic areas, then photocopy the relevant articles from the *BMJ* or the *BJGP* or, as aforementioned, you could utilise the Internet.

▶ Assuming you have a group of five candidates, then give each candidate four of the top twenty topic areas to study. Set yourselves a target of, say 4 weeks maximum, to produce;
  – a precis of the articles.
  – copies of the full articles.

It would also be helpful for each candidate to produce a one-paragraph statement about the relevance of the specific hot topic.

Perennial hot topics

My suggested list is as follows:

Ethical dilemmas
Your revision should include the following areas:

▶ Confidentiality. Read the General Medical Council *Duties of a Doctor*, and consider your role as a GP in maintaining confidentiality about your patients and partners. Know about when you can ethically breach confidentiality; the old chestnut here is the epileptic driver who refuses to advise DVLA of his medical condition.

▶ The alcoholic partner and the effect that it is having on patients and partners in the practice.

▶ Chaperones, and their role for both male and female GP.

▶ Living wills. Advance directives, including medico-legal aspects of these.

▶ Euthanasia. Although it is illegal in the UK, candidates are expected to have an opinion, particularly referring to the ethics of euthanasia within the European Union, e.g. in The Netherlands.

National guidelines for major conditions
Not only should you know the following guidelines in detail, but also have an opinion on them. Are these gold standards achievable? What are the implications, e.g. for maintaining a type 2 diabetic's blood pressure at 140/80 or less. Make clear the implications: to the patient in acceptability of drug treatment, including compliance and side-effect profiles, to the doctor and his practice, particularly involvement of medication in practice formularies and cost. Furthermore, study the implications for the practice team, specifically when you have a practice diabetic nurse, who clearly needs to be kept ahead of these recent developments.

▶ United Kingdom Prospective Diabetes Study – again are these gold standards achievable?

▶ British Hypertension Society Guidelines. These changed in 1999, with a lowering of the threshold for treatment.

▶ British Hypercholesterolaemia Guidelines. Compare these with Sheffield Guidelines.

▶ The British Guidelines on Asthma Management.

These guidelines are all readily available in MIMS magazine and, apart from taking photocopies, I would recommend that you individually put photocopies on your desk or on the wall in your consulting room, so you can readily refer to them when patients come in. In that way you utilise the guidelines during a consultation, and that makes them much easier to understand and learn from.

Revalidation/clinical governance/peer review/keeping up to date in general practice
All these topics are highly important at the turn of the millennium, and are likely to be for some years to come. You will not be expected just to accept that these may be taking place, but to have an opinion on them, e.g. in revalidation and the potential costs involved, and who is going to bear these costs. What are the implications for GPs

who fail their revalidation? Who needs to pay for their retraining? When do they get referred to the General Medical Council? Is the General Medical Council the appropriate body to whom these individuals should be referred?

Depression
All GPs realise that depression is an increasing problem, and patients are much more pro-active now in coming forward if they are depressed. The Defeat Depression Campaign of the 1990s has great relevance. No candidate should enter the MRCGP examination without an in-depth understanding of depression, its presentation, the effects on the family, and the debate regarding appropriate and cost-effective medication.

Evidence-based general practice
This is here to stay, and again candidates will be expected to give an opinion on the pros and cons of this.

Complaints procedures
Although practices are expected to have an in-house complaints procedure as advised by the Health Authority, candidates should have an understanding of how these procedures run, and may be asked in an examination to give an example of a complaint they have heard of, or have been involved with.

Coronary heart disease
As always, this is highly topical.

Teenage health
As aforementioned, this comes up over and over again in the *BMJ* and the *BJGP*, and is clearly an area which can cause concern with candidates, particularly as in some areas teenagers feel that their health is not being appropriately addressed by GPs. Does your practice have a protocol for dealing with teenage health, or does the practice have a teenage health clinic? What is your own attitude towards teenage health?

Stress management and burn out
In my experience as a College Examiner, candidates in the Orals often appear very surprised when you ask them what their own personal stress management protocol is, and how they would avoid burn out!

Personal protection
Be aware of ways of protecting yourself when on call, and your obligations regarding the drugs you carry.

Premises
This topic is often overlooked by candidates, but is indeed a very important topic area, particularly regarding your obligations under Health and Safety at Work and COSHH regulations.

Practice staff

Again an area often overlooked by candidates; you should be aware of the employment law with regard to your staff. Questions frequently come up on how to employ new staff.

Screening

Understand Wilson's criteria, and their application to e.g. national mammography service and cervical screening. Understand the difference between screening and surveillance.

Audit

Have a full understanding of exactly what audit means, and be prepared to give some examples. You may even get an audit in the written paper to comment on, and it is highly likely that questions on audit will come up in the oral examinations.

Summary

It is hoped that this short chapter will act as a catalyst in assisting you to spot hot topics. Previous experience of candidates following this method has shown that many candidates are pleasantly surprised when they find that several of the hot topic areas they have prepared have actually come up in examination.

Index